Oxford
Handbook of
Endocrinology and
Diabetes

Oxford Handbook of Endocrinology and Diabetes

Helen E Turner

and

John A H Wass

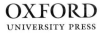

OXFORD
UNIVERSITY PRESS

Great Clarendon Street, Oxford OX2 6DP

Oxford University Press is a department of the University of Oxford.
It furthers the University's objective of excellence in research, scholarship,
and education by publishing worldwide in

Oxford New York

Auckland Bangkok Buenos Aires Cape Town Chennai
Dar es Salaam Delhi Hong Kong Istanbul Karachi Kolkata
Kuala Lumpur Madrid Melbourne Mexico City Mumbai Nairobi
São Paulo Shanghai Taipei Tokyo Toronto

Oxford is a registered trade mark of Oxford University Press
in the UK and in certain other countries

Published in the United States
by Oxford University Press Inc., New York

© Oxford University Press, 2002

The moral rights of the authors have been asserted
Database right Oxford University Press (maker)

First published 2002
Servier edn. printed 2003

A catalogue record for this title is available from the British Library

Library of Congress Cataloging in Publication Data

Oxford handbook of endocrinology and diabetes / edited by Helen E. Turner and
John A. H. Wass.
1. Endocrinology—Handbooks, manuals, etc.   2. Diabetes—Handbooks, manuals,
etc. I. Turner, Helen, 1967–. II. Wass, John.
RC649.O96 2001   616.4—dc21   2001052102

ISBN 0 19 263052 0
ISBN 0 19 853070 6 Part 1 (Servier edn.)
ISBN 0 19 853077 3 Part 2 (Servier edn.)

10 9 8 7 6 5 4 3 2 1

Typeset by EXPO Holdings, Malaysia
Printed in Italy by LegoPrint S.p.A.

Preface

Our aim with this handbook is to provide a readily assimilable 'white coat pocket' book in endocrinology and diabetes, which is complementary to the *Oxford Textbook of Endocrinology and Diabetes*. Our target audience is trainees and also the trained who may have the occasional mental blank.

We are grateful to our contributors for their excellent and timely efforts and we are particularly grateful to Richard Sheaves for his considerable help in planning the book.

We have necessarily been didactic, but in order to minimize the effects of personal idiosyncrasies, we have sent each chapter to two external referees. Their names are recorded elsewhere. We are very grateful indeed to this panel of experts and for the enormous trouble that they have taken in going through the manuscript with the utmost care.

We regard this volume as the start of an evolutionary process and the first of many editions. We encourage readers to write with constructive comments and suggestions.

Helen Turner
John Wass
Department of Endocrinology
Oxford Centre for Diabetes, Endocrinology and Metabolism
Radcliffe Infirmary
Oxford
UK

March 2002

Acknowledgements

We would like to record our sincere thanks to the following friends and colleagues for their review and advice on various sections:

Professor A B Atkinson, Metabolic Unit, Royal Victoria Hospital, Belfast

Dr JS Bevan, Department of Endocrinology, Aberdeen Royal Infirmary, Aberdeen

Dr P M Bouloux, Department of Endocrinology, Royal Free Hospital, London

Dr P E Clayton, Department of Child Health, Royal Manchester Children's Hospital, Manchester

Dr G S Conway, Cobbold Laboratories, Middlesex Hospital, London

Dr N Finer, Department of Endocrinology, Luton and Dunstable Hospital, Luton

Professor J A Franklyn, Department of Medicine, Queen Elizabeth Hospital, Birmingham

Professor S Franks, Department of Endocrinology, St Mary's Hospital Medical School, London

Professor AB Grossman, Department of Endocrinology, St Bartholomew's Hospital, London

Professor R R Holman, Diabetes Trials Unit, Oxford Centre for Diabetes, Endocrinology and Metabolism, Radcliffe Infirmary, Oxford

Professor D Hosking, Division of Mineral Medicine, City Hospital, Nottingham

Dr D R Matthews, Oxford Centre for Diabetes, Endocrinology and Metabolism, Radcliffe Infirmary, Oxford

Dr A Neil, Oxford Centre for Diabetes, Endocrinology and Metabolism, Radcliffe Infirmary, Oxford

Professor CWG Redman, Nuffield Department of Obstetrics and Gynaecology, John Radcliffe Hospital, Oxford

Professor M O Savage, Department of Paediatric Endocrinology, St Bartholomew's Hospital, London

Dr B Shine, Department of Biochemistry, John Radcliffe Hospital, Oxford

Professor PM Stewart, Department of Medicine, Queen Elizabeth Hospital, Edgbaston, Birmingham

Professor R Thakker, Nuffield Department of Medicine, John Radcliffe Hospital, Oxford and Oxford Centre for Diabetes, Endocrinology and Metabolism, Radcliffe Infirmary, Oxford

Professor A P Weetman, Clinical Science Centre, Northern General Hospital, Sheffield

Professor F Wu, Department of Endocrinology, Manchester Royal Infirmary, Manchester.

Contents

Foreword

In this day and age of the internet, multimedia materials, and interactive CDs it is easy to forget that old-fashioned method of learning and education – the book. I suspect that many like myself still prefer to look things up in a book rather than wrestle with a computer. There are two main types of book – the reference book and the handy manual. The former is useful when you wish to review a topic in depth or look up an uncommon condition or presentation, but often one wants to check a simple detail, for example a reference range or diagnostic criterion. Handbooks are ideal for this as they can be carried around or kept easily available. The current work is an ideal example. It is packed with useful information and is very up to date – something not shared by most major textbooks. It is ideally suited for the specialist registrar in endocrinology and diabetes – and even more so for the ageing consultant. It will also be useful in general practice with specific regard to the diabetes and thyroid sections. This is extremely important with the development of primary care diabetes clinics and the explosive rise in prevalence of diabetes, particularly in non-Europeans. It contains many helpful practical nuggets and will, I am sure, be required briefcase or pocket content. It fills a gap in an important area of clinical practice. The authors and publishers are to be commended – I just hope that the next edition has already been planned.

Professor Sir George Alberti
President
Royal College of Physicians
London, UK

Contributors

David B Dunger Department of Paediatrics, University of Cambridge, Cambridge, UK

Mohgah Elsheikh Department of Diabetes and Endocrinology, Royal Berkshire Hospital, Reading, Berkshire, UK

Ken Ong Department of Paediatrics, University of Cambridge, Cambridge, UK

Mahesh Sathiavageeswaran Department of Endocrinology, Oxford Centre for Diabetes, Endocrinology and Metabolism, Radcliffe Infirmary, Oxford OX2 6HE, UK

Barry M Seemungal Department of Endocrinology, Oxford Centre for Diabetes, Endocrinology and Metabolism, Radcliffe Infirmary, Oxford OX2 6HE, UK

Peter Selby Department of Medicine, Manchester Royal Infirmary, Oxford Road, Manchester M13 9WL, UK

Richard Sheaves Division of Medicine, Jersey Hospital, Jersey, Channel Islands

Kevin P Shotliff Department of Medicine, Kingston Hospital, Kingston upon Thames, Surrey KT2 7QB, UK

Garry D Tan Oxford Centre for Diabetes, Endocrinology and Metabolism, Radcliffe Infirmary, Oxford OX2 6HE, UK

Helen E Turner Department of Endocrinology, Oxford Centre for Diabetes, Endocrinology and Metabolism, Radcliffe Infirmary, Oxford OX2 6HE, UK

John A H Wass Department of Endocrinology, Oxford Centre for Diabetes, Endocrinology and Metabolism, Radcliffe Infirmary, Oxford OX2 6HE, UK

H John Wong Department of Clinical Biochemistry, Kingston Hospital, Kingston upon Thames, Surrey KT2 7QB, UK

Abbreviations

ACE	angiotensin converting enzyme
ACEI	angiotensin converting enzyme inhibitor
AD	autosomal dominant
ADA	American Diabetes Association
ADH	antidiuretic hormone
AGE	advanced glycation end-products
AIH	amiodarone-induced hypothyroidism
AIT	amiodarone-induced thyrotoxicosis
ALT	alanine transaminase
ANP	atrial natriuretic peptide
ART	assisted reproductive techniques
AST	aspartate transaminase
ATD	antithyroid drug
BMD	bone mineral density
BP	blood pressure
CaE	calcium excretion
CAH	congenital adrenal hyperplasia
CBG	cortisol binding globulin
CHD	coronary heart disease
CMV	cytomegalovirus
CPA	cyproterone acetate
CRF	chronic renal failure
CRH	corticotrophin releasing hormone
CSF	cerebrospinal fluid
CSII	continuous subcutaneous insulin infusion
CSW	cerebral salt wasting syndrome
CT	computed tomography
CVP	central venous pressure
DCCT	Diabetes Control and Complications Trial
DCT	distal convolutued tubule
DHEA	dihydroepiandrostenedione

DHT	dihydrotestosterone
DI	diabetes insipidus
DIDMOAD	*di*abetes *i*nsipidus, *DM*, *o*ptic *a*trophy + sensorineural *d*eafness (Wolfram's syndrome)
DVLA	Driver and Vehicle Licensing Agency
DVT	deep vein thrombosis
DXA	dual energy X-ray absorptiometry
EE2	ethinyl oestradiol
ESR	erythrocyte sedimentation rate
ESRF	end-stage renal failure
ETDRS	Early Treatment of Diabetic Retinopathy Study
FBC	full blood count
FCHL	familial combined hyperlipidaemia
FDB	familial defective apolipoprotein B-100
FH	familial hypercholesterolaemia
FHH	familial hypocalciuric hypercalcaemia
FNAC	fine needle aspiration cytology
FSH	follicle stimulating hormone
FTC	follicular carcinoma
GAD	glutamic acid decarboxylase
GFR	glomerular filtration rate
GH	growth hormone
GHD	growth hormone deficiency
GI	gastrointestinal
GIFT	gamete intrafallopian transfer
GIP	gastric inhibitory peptide
GRTH	generalized resistance to thyroid hormone
hCG	human chorionic gonadotrophin
HDL	high-density lipoprotein
5HIAA	5-hydroxyindole acetic acid
HLA	human leukocyte antigens
HMG CoA	3-hydroxy-3-methylglutaryl coenzyme A
HNF	hepatic nuclear factor
HPA	hypothalmic–pituitary–adrenal (axis)
HSG	hysterosalpingography
HZV	herpes zoster virus
ICSI	intracytoplasmic sperm injection

IDDM	insulin dependent diabetes mellitus (type 1)
IDL	intermediate-density lipoprotein
IFG	impaired fasting hyperglycaemia
IGF-I	insulin-like growth factor-1
IGT	impaired glucose tolerance
IHH	idiopathic hypogonadotrophic hypogonadism
IPSS	inferior petrosal sinus sampling
IRMA	intraretinal microvascular abnormalities
ITT	insulin tolerance test
IU	international units
IUGR	intrauterine growth retardation
IUI	intrauterine insemination
IVF	*in vitro* fertilization
KS	Kaposi sarcoma
LCAT	lecithin : cholesterol acyltransferase
LDL	low-density lipoprotein
LFT	liver function test
LH	luteinizing hormone
MAI	Mycobacterium avium intracellulare
MC	mineralocorticoid
MEN	multiple endocrine neoplasia
MHC	major histocompatibility complex
MI	myocardial infarct
MIBG	^{123}Iodine-metaiodobenzylguanidine
MIS	mullerian inhibitory substance
MODY	maturity onset diabetes of the young
MPH	mid-parental height
MRSA	methicillin-resistant *Staphylococcus aureus*
MTC	medullary thyroid cancer
NF	neurofibromatosis
NFA	non-functioning pituitary adenoma
NGF	nerve growth factor
NICH	non-islet cell hypoglycaemia
NIDDM	non-insulin dependent diabetes mellitus (type 2)
NVD	new vessels on the disc (diabetic retinopathy)
NVE	new vessels elsewhere (diabetic retinopathy)
OCP	oral contraceptive pill

OGTT	oral glucose tolerance test
25OHD	25-hydroxy vitamin D
17OHP	17-hydroxyprogesterone
OHSS	ovarian hyperstimulation syndrome
PAI	platelet activator inhibitor
PCOS	polycystic ovary syndrome
PCT	postcoital test
PET	positron emission spectrography
PID	pelvic inflammatory disease
PIH	pregnancy-induced hypertension
PMC	papillary microcarcinoma of the thyroid
PNMT	phenylethanolamine-N-methyl transferase
POF	premature ovarian failure
POMC	pro-opiomelanocortin
PP	pancreatic polypeptide
PPAR	peroxisome proliferator activated receptor
PRL	prolactin
PRTH	pituitary resistance to thyroid hormones
PSA	prostatic specific antigen
PTH	parathyroid hormone
PTHrP	parathyroid hormone related peptide
QALY	Quality Adjusted Life Year
QCT	quantitative computed tomography
QUS	quantitative ultrasound
SHBG	sex hormone binding globulin
T_3	tri-iodothyronine
T_4	thyroxine
TB	tuberculosis
TBG	T_4-binding globulin
TBPA	T_4-binding prealbumin
TFT	thyroid function test
TG	triglycerides
TGF	transforming growth factor
TNF	tumour necrosis factor
TPO	thyroid peroxidase
TRH	thyrotropin releasing hormone
TSAb	TSH stimulating antibodies

TSG	tumour suppressor genes
TSH	thyroid stimulating hormone
TSH-RAB	TSH receptor antibodies
TTR	transthyretin
U&Es	urea and electolytes
UFC	urinary free cortisol
UKPDS	UK Prospective Diabetes Study
VEGF	vascular endothelial growth factor
VHL	Von Hippel–Lindau disease
VIP	vasoactive intestinal peptide
VLDL	very high-density lipoprotein
WDHA	watery diarrhoea, hypokalaemia, and achlorhydria
WHO	World Health Organization
ZE	Zollinger Ellison syndrome

Part I
Thyroid

Chapter 1
Anatomy and physiology of the thyroid

Anatomy

The thyroid gland comprises
- a midline isthmus lying horizontally just below the cricoid cartilage
- two lateral lobes that extend upward over the lower half of the thyroid cartilage.

The gland lies deep to the strap muscles of the neck, enclosed in the pre-tracheal fascia, which anchors it to the trachea, so that the thyroid moves up on swallowing.

Histology

- Fibrous septa divide the gland into pseudolobules.
- Pseudolobules are composed of vesicles called follicles or acini, surrounded by a capillary network.
- The follicle walls are lined by cuboidal epithelium.
- The lumen is filled with a proteinaceous colloid, which contains the unique protein thyroglobulin. The peptide sequences of T_4 and T_3 are synthesized and stored as a component of thyroglobulin.

Development

- Develops from the endoderm of the floor of the pharynx with some contribution from the lateral pharyngeal pouches.
- Descent of the midline thyroid anlage gives rise to the thyroglossal duct, which extends from the foramen caecum near the base of the tongue to the isthmus of the thyroid.
- During development the posterior aspect of the thyroid becomes associated with the parathyroid gland and the parafollicular C cells, derived from the ultimo-branchial body, which become incorporated into its substance.
- The C cells are the source of calcitonin and give rise to medullary thyroid carcinoma when they undergo malignant transformation.
- The foetal thyroid begins to concentrate and organify iodine at about 10–12 weeks gestation.
- Maternal TRH readily crosses the placenta, maternal TSH and T_4 do not.
- T_4 from the foetal thyroid is the major thyroid hormone available to the foetus. The foetal pituitary–thyroid axis is a functional unit distinct from that of the mother.

Thyroid examination

Inspection

• Look at the neck from the front. If a goitre (enlarged thyroid gland of whatever cause) is present, the patient should be asked to swallow. Goitre moves up with swallowing.

• Watch for appearance of any nodule not visible before swallowing, e.g. retrosternal goitre in the elderly.

Palpation

• Is the thyroid gland tender to touch?

• With index and middle finger feel below thyroid cartilage where the isthmus of the thyroid gland lies over the trachea.

• Palpate the two lobes of the thyroid, which extend laterally behind the sternomastoid muscle.

• Ask the patient to swallow again while you continue to palpate the thyroid.

• Assess *size*, whether it is *soft*, firm *or hard*, it is *nodular* or *diffusely* enlarged and whether it *moves* readily on swallowing.

• Palpate along the medial edge of the sternomastoid muscle on either side to look for a pyramidal lobe.

• Palpate for lymph nodes

Percussion

• Percuss upper mediastinum for retrosternal goitre.

Auscultation

• Auscultate to identify bruits, consistent with Graves' disease.

• Occasionally inspiratory stridor can be heard with a large or retrosternal goitre causing tracheal compression.

Assess thyroid status

• Observe for signs of thyroid disease – exophthalmos, proptosis, thyroid acropachy, pretibial myxoedema, hyperactivity, restlessness, or whether immobile and uninterested.

• Take pulse; note presence or absence of tachycardia, bradycardia or atrial fibrillation.

• Feel palms – whether warm and sweaty or cold.

• Look for tremor in outstretched arms.

• Examine eyes:
exophthalmos (sclera visible above lower lid); lid retraction: sclera visible above cornea; lid lag; conjuctivitis; periorbital oedema; loss of full-range movement

Physiology

- Thyroid hormone contains iodine. Iodine enters the thyroid in the form of inorganic or ionic iodide, which is oxidized by a peroxidase enzyme at the cell–colloid interface. Subsequent reactions result in the formation of iodothyronines.

- The thyroid is the only source of T_4.

- The thyroid secretes 20% of T_3; the remainder is generated in extraglandular tissues by the conversion of T_4 to T_3.

Synthesis of the thyroid hormones can be inhibited by a variety of agents termed *goitrogens*.

- Perchlorate and thiocyanate inhibit iodide transport

- Thioureas and mercaptoimidazole inhibit the initial oxidation of iodide and coupling of iodothyronines.

- In large doses iodine itself blocks organic binding and coupling reactions.

- Lithium has several inhibitory effects on intrathyroidal iodine metabolism.

In the blood, T_4 and T_3 are almost entirely bound to plasma proteins. T_4 is bound in decreasing order of intensity to T_4 binding globulin (TBG), transthyretin (TTR), and albumin. T_3 is bound 10–20 times less firmly by TBG and not significantly by TTR. Only the free or unbound hormone is available to tissues. The metabolic state correlates more closely with the free than the total hormone concentration in the plasma. The relatively weak binding of T_3 accounts for its more rapid onset and offset of action. Table 1.1 summarizes those states associated with primary alterations in the concentration of TBG. When there is primarily an alteration in the concentration of thyroid hormones, the concentration of TBG changes little (Table 1.2).

Concentration of free hormones does not vary directly with that of the total hormones; e.g. while the total T_4 level rises in pregnancy, the free T_4 level remains normal.

The levels of thyroid hormone in the blood are tightly controlled by feedback mechanisms involved in the hypothalamo–pituitary–thyroid axis (Fig. 1.1).

- TSH secreted by the pituitary stimulates the thyroid to secrete principally T_4 and also T_3. TRH stimulates the synthesis and secretion of TSH. T_4 and T_3 inhibit TSH synthesis and secretion directly.

Table 1.1 Disordered thyroid hormone–protein interactions

	Serum total T_4 and T_3	Free T_4 and T_3
Primary abnormality in TBG		
▲Concentration	↑	Normal
▼Concentration	↓	Normal
Primary disorder of thyroid function		
Hyperthyroidism	↑	↑
Hypothyroidism	↓	↓

- T_4 and T_3 are bound to TBG, TTR, and albumin. The remaining free hormones inhibit synthesis and release of TRH to influence growth and metabolism.

Table 1.2 Circumstances associated with altered concentration of TBG

Increased TBG	Decreased TBG
Pregnancy	Androgens
Newborn state	Large doses of glucocorticoids; Cushings' syndrome
OCP and other sources of oestrogens	Chronic liver disease
Tamoxifen	Severe systemic illness
Hepatitis A; chronic active hepatitis	Active acromegaly
Biliary cirrhosis	Nephrotic syndrome
Acute intermittent porphyria	Genetically determined
Genetically determined	Drugs, e.g. phenytoin

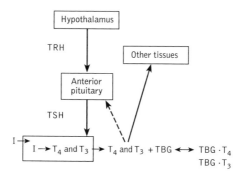

Fig. 1.1 Regulation of thyroid function. Solid arrows indicate stimulation, broken arrow indicates inhibitory influence. TRH, thyrotropin releasing hormone; TSH, thyroid stimulating hormone; T_4, thyroxine; T_3, tri-iodothyronine; I, iodine; TBG, thyroid binding globulin.

- T_4 is converted peripherally to the metabolically active T_3 or the inactive reverse T_3 (rT_3).
- T_4 and T_3 are metabolized in the liver by conjugation with glucuronate and sulfate. Enzyme inducers such as phenobarbital, carbamazepine, and phenytoin increase the metabolic clearance of the hormones without decreasing the proportion of free hormone in the blood.

Abnormalities of development

- Remnants of the thyroglossal duct may be found in any position along the course of the tract of its descent:
  - in the tongue, it is referred to as '*lingual thyroid*'
  - *thyroglossal cysts* may be visible as midline swellings in the neck
  - *thyroglossal fistula* develops an opening in the middle of the neck.
  - *thyroglossal nodules* or
  - the '*pyramidal lobe*', a structure contiguous with the thyroid isthmus which extends upwards.
- The gland can descend too far down to reach the anterior mediastinum.
- Congenital hypothyroidism results from failure of the thyroid to develop.

Chapter 2
Thyroid investigations

Tests of hormone concentration

(Table 2.1)

Highly specific and sensitive radioimmunoassays are used to measure serum T4 and T3 concentrations. Free hormone concentrations usually correlate better with the metabolic state than do total hormone concentrations because they are unaffected by changes in binding protein concentration or affinity.

Tests of homeostatic control

• Serum TSH concentration is used as first line in the diagnosis of primary hypothyroidism and hyperthyroidism. The test is misleading in patients with secondary thyroid dysfunction.

• The TRH stimulation test, which can be used to assess the functional state of the TSH secretory mechanism, is now rarely used to diagnose primary thyroid disease since it has been superseded by sensitive TSH assays. It is of limited use; its main use is in the differential diagnosis of elevated TSH in the setting of elevated thyroid hormone levels.

In interpreting results of TFTs, the effects of drugs that the patient might be on should be borne in mind. Table 2.2 lists the influence of drugs on TFTs.

Table 2.1 Thyroid hormone concentrations in various thyroid abnormalities

Condition	TSH	Free T$_4$	Free T$_3$
Primary hyperthyroidism	Undetectable	↑↑	↑
T$_3$ toxicosis	Undetectable	Normal	↑↑
Subclinical hyperthyroidism	↓	Normal	Normal
Secondary hyperthyroidism (TSHoma)	↑ or normal	↑	↑
Thyroid hormone resistance	↑ or normal	↑	↑
Primary hypothyroidism	↑	↓	↓ or normal
Secondary hypothyroidism	↓ or normal	↓	↓ or normal

Thyroid hormone resistance (RTH)

+ Syndrome characterized by reduced responsiveness to elevated circulating levels of free T_4 and free T_3, non-suppressed serum TSH and intact TSH responsiveness to TRH. Clinical features may be absent but may include short stature, hyperactivity, attention deficits with mental deficiency or learning disability, and goitre.

+ Differential diagnosis includes TSH-secreting pituitary tumour.

+ Treatment depending on clinical features is to supplement thyroid hormone, depending on parameters of tissue responses to thyroid hormone. See page 47.

Table 2.2 Influence of drugs on thyroid function tests

Metabolic process	Increased	Decreased
TSH secretion	Amiodarone (transiently: becomes normal after 2–3 months)	Glucocorticoids, dopamine agonists, phenytoin, dopamine
T_4 synthesis/ release	Iodide	Iodide, lithium
Binding proteins	Oestrogen, clofibrate, heroin	Glucocorticoids, androgens, phenytoin, carbamazepine
T_4 metabolism	Anticonvulsants; rifampicin	
T_4/T_3 binding in serum		Salicylates, frusemide, mefenamic acid, amiodarone, ß-blockers, glucocorticoids

Table 2.3 Atypical thyroid function tests

Test	Possible cause
Suppressed TSH and normal free T_4	T_3 toxicosis (approximately 5% of thyrotoxicosis)
Suppressed TSH and normal free T_4 and free T_3	Early subclinical thyrotoxicosis Recovery from thyrotoxicosis Excess thyroxine replacement Sick euthyroidism
Detectable TSH and elevated free T_4 and free T_3	TSH secreting pituitary tumour Thyroid hormone resistance Heterophile antibodies
Elevated free T_4 and low free T_3	Amiodarone

Antibody screen (Table 2.4)

High titres of antithyroid peroxidase (Anti TPO) antibodies or antithyroglobulin antibodies are found in patients with autoimmune thyroid disease (Hashimoto's thyroiditis; Graves' disease)

Table 2.4 Antithyroid antibodies and thyroid disease

Condition	Anti-TPO	Anti-thyroglobulin	TSH receptor antibody
Graves' disease	70–80%	30–50%	70–100% (stimulating)
Autoimmune hypothyroidism	Majority	Majority	10–20% (blocking)

Note: TSH receptor antibodies may be stimulatory or inhibitory.

Screening for thyroid disease

The following categories of patients should be screened for thyroid disease:

- patients with atrial fibrillation or hyperlipidaemia
- periodic (6 monthly) assessments in patients receiving amiodarone and lithium
- annual check of thyroid function in the annual review of diabetic patients
- women with type 1 diabetes in the first trimester of pregnancy and post delivery (because of the threefold rise in incidence of postpartum thyroid dysfunction in such patients)
- women with past history of postpartum thyroiditis
- annual check of thyroid function in people with Down's syndrome, Turner's syndrome and Addison's disease, in view of the high prevalence of hypothyroidism in such patients.

(WM Tunbridge and MP Vanderpump; *Endocrinology and Metabolism Clinics of North America* 2000; 29(2): 239–253)

Scintiscanning

Permits localization of sites of accumulation of radioiodine or sodium pertechnetate [^{99m}Tc], which gives information about the activity of the iodine trap (Table 2.5). This is useful:

+ to define areas of increased or decreased function within the thyroid (Table 2.6) which occasionally helps in cases of uncertainty as to the cause of the thyrotoxicosis
+ to detect retrosternal goitre
+ to detect ectopic thyroid tissue
+ to detect functioning metastases of thyroid carcinoma.

Agents which influence thyroid uptake, including

+ intake of high-iodine foods, such as kelp (seaweed)
+ drugs containing iodine, such as amiodarone
+ recent use of radiographic contrast dyes

can potentially interfere with the interpretation of the scan.

Table 2.5 Radioisotope scans

	^{123}Iodine	^{99}Technitium pertechnetate
Half-life	Short	Short
Advantage	Low emission of radiation Have higher energy photons. Hence useful for imaging a toxic goitre with a substernal component	Maximum thyroid uptake within 30 min of administration. Can be used in breast-feeding women (discontinue feeding for 24 h)
Disadvantage		Technetium is only trapped by the thyroid without being organified
Use	Functional assessment of the thyroid	Rapid scanning

Table 2.6 Radionuclide scanning (scintigram) in thyroid disease

Condition	Scan appearance
Graves' hyperthyroidism	Enlarged gland Increased homogeneous radionucleotide uptake
Thyroiditis (e.g. de Quervains)	Low or absent uptake
Toxic nodule	A solitary area of high uptake
Thyrotoxicosis factitia	Depressed thyroid uptake
Thyroid cancer	Successful ^{131}I uptake by tumour tissue requires an adequate level of TSH, achieved by stopping T_3 replacement 10 days before scanning or giving recombinant TSH injection

Ultrasound scanning

Provides an accurate indication of size and is useful for differentiating cystic nodules from solid ones, but cannot be used to distinguish between benign and malignant disease.

• Microcalcification within nodules favours the diagnosis of malignancy; micro-calcifications smaller than 2 mm in diameter are observed in ~60% of malignant nodules, but in <2% of benign lesions.

• Calcification is a prominent feature of medullary carcinoma of the thyroid.

• It can detect whether a nodule is solitary or part of a multinodular process.

• Sequential scanning can be employed to assess changes in size of thyroid over time.

Note Neither scintigraphy or ultrasound is routinely indicated in a patient with goitre.

Fine needle aspiration cytology

- FNAC is now considered the most accurate test for diagnosis of thyroid nodules. It is performed in an outpatient setting. 2–4 aspirations are carried out at different sites for each nodule. Cytologic findings are *satisfactory* or *diagnostic* in approximately 85% of specimens and *non-diagnostic* in the remainder.
- In experienced hands FNAC is an excellent diagnostic technique, as shown in the table below.
- Repeat FNAC after 3–6 months further reduces the proportion of false negatives.
- It is impossible to differentiate between benign and malignant follicular neoplasm using FNAC. Therefore surgical excision of a follicular neoplasm is always indicated.

Feature	Range (%)	Mean Value(%)
Accuracy	85–100	95
Specificity	72–100	92
Sensitivity	65–98	83
False negative	1–11	5

Computed tomography (CT)

- CT is useful in the evaluation of retrosternal and retrotracheal extension of an enlarged thyroid.
- Compression of the trachea and displacement of the major vessels can be identified with CT of the superior mediastinum.
- It can demonstrate the extent of intrathoracic extension of thyroid malignancy and infiltration of adjacent structures such as the carotid artery, internal jugular vein, trachea, oesophagus and regional lymph nodes.

Additional laboratory investigations

Haematological tests

• Long-standing thyrotoxicosis may be associated with a *normo-chromic anaemia* and occasionally a *mild neutropenia, lymphocytosis* and rarely a *thrombocytopenia*.

• In hypothyroidism a *macrocytosis* is typical, although concurrent vitamin B_{12} deficiency should be considered.

• There may also be a *microcytic anaemia* due to menorrhagia and impaired iron utilization.

Biochemical tests

• *Alkaline phosphatase* may be elevated.

• Mild *hypercalcaemia* occasionally occurs in thyrotoxicosis and reflects increased bone resorption. *Hypercalcuria* is more common.

• In a hypothyroid patient, *hyponatraemia* may be due to reduced renal tubular loss or less commonly due to co-existing cortisol deficiency.

• In hypothyroidism *creatinine kinase* is often raised and the lipid profile altered with *increased LDL cholesterol.*

Endocrine tests

• In hypothyroidism, serum *prolactin* may be elevated because increased TRH leads to increased prolactin secretion.

• In thyrotoxicosis there is an increase in *sex hormone binding globulin (SHBG)*, and a complex interaction with sex steroid hormone metabolism, resulting in changes in the levels of androgens and oestrogens. The net physiological result is an increase in *oestrogenic* activity, with *gynaecomastia* and a decrease in libido in men presenting with thyrotoxicosis.

Sick euthyroid syndrome (Non thyroidal illness syndrome)

- Biochemistry – Low T4 and T3
  – Inappropriately normal/suppressed TSH
- Tissue thyroid hormone concentrations are very low
- Context – Starvation
  – Severe illness eg ITU, severe infections, renal failure, cardiac failure, liver failure, end-stage malignancy
- Whether replacement thyroxine treatment provides benefit is unclear.

Atypical clinical situations

- *Thyrotoxicosis factitia*
  - no thyroid enlargement
  - elevated free T_4 and suppressed TSH
  - depressed thyroid uptake on scintigraphy
  - low thyroglobulin differentiates from thyroiditis (which shows depressed uptake on scintigraphy but increased thyroglobulin) and all other causes of elevated thyroid hormones.
- *Struma ovarii* (ovarian teratoma containing hyperfunctioning thyroid tissue):
  - no thyroid enlargement
  - depressed thyroid uptake on scintigraphy
  - body scan after radioiodine confirms diagnosis.
- *Trophoblast tumours* hCG has structural homology with TSH and leads to thyroid gland stimulation, and usually mild thyrotoxicosis.
- *Hyperemesis gravidarum* Thyroid function tests may be abnormal with a suppressed TSH (See Chapter 70 on thyroid disorders and pregnancy).
- *Choriocarcinoma of the testes* may be associated with gynaecomastia and thyrotoxicosis – measure hCG.

Chapter 3
Thyrotoxicosis

Aetiology

Epidemiology

- 10 times more common in women than in men in the UK.
- Prevalence is approximately 2% of the female population.
- Annual incidence is 3 cases per 1000 women.

Definition of thyrotoxicosis and hyperthyroidism

- The term *thyrotoxicosis* denotes the clinical, physiological, and biochemical findings that result when the tissues are exposed to excess thyroid hormone. It can arise in a variety of ways (Table 3.1). It is essential to establish a specific diagnosis as this determines therapy choices and provides important information for the patient regarding prognosis.
- The term *hyperthyroidism* should be used to denote only those conditions in which hyperfunction of the thyroid leads to thyrotoxicosis.

Genetics of Graves' disease

- Graves' disease is a complex autoimmune disorder. Genes make only a moderate contribution to susceptibility.
- Several genetic susceptibility loci and environmental factors are likely to contribute to the development of the disease
- HLA-DR3, HLA-DQA1*0501, and the *CTLA-4* (cytotoxic T lymphocyte associated-4) gene region have been established as susceptibility loci; HLA-DQA1*0701 protects against Graves' disease.
- Additional loci are likely to be identified via a combination of genome-wide linkage analysis and allelic association analysis of candidate genes.

Table 3.1 Classification of the aetiology of thyrotoxicosis

Associated with hyperthyroidism	
Excessive thyroid stimulation	Graves' disease, Hashitoxicosis
	Pituitary thyrotroph adenoma
	Pituitary thyroid hormone resistance syndrome (excess TSH)
	Trophoblastic tumours producing hCG with thyrotrophic activity
Thyroid nodules with autonomous function	Toxic solitary nodule, toxic multinodular goiter
	Very rarely, thyroid cancer
Not associated with hyperthyroidism	
Thyroid inflammation	Silent and postpartum thyroiditis, subacute (de Quervain's) thyroiditis
	Drug-induced thyroiditis (amiodarone)
Exogenous thyroid hormones	Overtreatment with thyroid hormone
	Thyrotoxicosis factitia (thyroxine use in non-thyroidal disease)
Ectopic thyroid tissue	Metastatic thyroid carcinoma
	Struma ovarii (teratoma containing functional thyroid tissue)

Manifestations of hyperthyroidism

Manifestations of hyperthyroidism (all forms)

Symptoms

- hyperactivity, irritability, altered mood, insomnia
- heat intolerance, increased sweating
- palpitations
- fatigue, weakness
- dyspnoea
- weight loss with increased appetite (weight gain in 10% of patients)
- pruritus
- increased stool frequency
- thirst and polyuria
- oligomenorrhoea or amenorrhoea, loss of libido

Signs

- sinus tachycardia, atrial fibrillation
- fine tremor, hyperkinesia, hyperreflexia
- warm, moist skin
- palmar erythema, onycholysis
- hair loss
- muscle weakness and wasting
- congestive (high output) heart failure, chorea, periodic paralysis (primarily in Asian men), psychosis (rare)

Investigation of thyrotoxicosis

- *Thyroid function tests* raised free T_4 and suppressed TSH (raised free T_3 in T_3 toxicosis)
- *Thyroid antibodies* see Table 2.4 (page 13).
- *Radionucleotide thyroid scan* if diagnosis uncertain (page 18).
- Thyrotoxic hypokalaemic periodic paralysis
  - Thyrotoxicosis
  - Potassium low
  - Intermittent muscle weakness + CPK ↑
  - Precipitated by heavy exertion or CHO load
  - Common in Asians

Manifestations of Graves' disease (in addition to the above)

* diffuse goitre
* ophthalmopathy (see p. 50)
  - a feeling of grittiness and discomfort in the eye
  - retrobulbar pressure or pain, eyelid lag or retraction
  - periorbital oedema, chemosis*, scleral injection*
  - exophthalmos (proptosis)*
  - extraocular muscle dysfunction*
  - exposure keratitis*
  - optic neuropathy*
* localized dermopathy (pretibial myxoedema p. 53)
* lymphoid hyperplasia
* thyroid acropachy (p. 53)

*Combination of these suggests congestive ophthalmopathy.

Urgent action necessary: if corneal ulceration, congestive ophthalmopathy, or optic neuropathy (p. 50).

Conditions associated with Graves' disease

* type 1 diabetes mellitus
* Addison's disease
* vitiligo
* pernicious anaemia
* alopecia areata
* myasthenia gravis
* coeliac disease
* other autoimmune disorders associated with the HLA-DR3 haplotype

Treatment

Medical treatment

In general, the standard policy in Europe is to offer a course of antithyroid drugs (ATD) first. In the USA, radioiodine is more likely to be offered as first-line treatment.

Aims and principles of medical treatment

- To induce remission in Graves' disease
- Monitor for relapse off treatment initially 6–8 weekly for 6 months, then 6 monthly for 2 years, and then annually thereafter or sooner if symptoms return.
- For relapse, consider definitive treatment such as radioiodine or surgery. A second course of ATD almost never results in remission.

Choice of drugs

- *Carbimazole*, which can be given as a single dose, is usually the drug of first choice in the UK.
- During pregnancy and lactation *propylthiouracil* is the drug of choice because of its lower concentration in breast milk and the possible association of carbimazole with aplasia cutis.
- 5 mg of carbimazole is roughly equivalent to 50 mg of propylthiouracil. Propylthiouracil has a theoretical advantage of inhibiting the conversion of T_4 to T_3, and T_3 levels decline more rapidly after starting the drug.
- 30–40 % of patients treated with an ATD remain euthyroid 10 years after discontinuation of therapy. If hyperthyroidism recurs after treatment with an ATD, there is little chance that a second course of treatment will result in permanent remission. Young patients, those with large goitres, ophthalmopathy, or high serum concentrations of thyrotropin receptor antibody at the time of diagnosis are unlikely to have a permanent remission.
- *β-Adrenergic antagonists* Propranolol 20–80 mg 3× daily. Considerable relief from such symptoms as anxiety, tremor, and palpitations may be gained in the initial 4–8 weeks of treatment.

Side-effects

- ATDs are generally well tolerated. Uncommonly, patients may complain of gastrointestinal symptoms or an alteration in their sense of taste and smell.

Treatment regimes

Two alternative regimes are practised: dose titration and block and replace.

Dose titration regime

- The primary aim is to achieve euthyroid state with high drug doses and then to maintain euthyroidism with a low stable dose. The dose of carbimazole or propylthiouracil is titrated according to the thyroid function tests performed every 4–8 weeks, aiming for a detectable TSH in the normal range. If free T_3 is >6 pmol/L carbimazole is started at 40 mg and if free T_3 is <6 pmol/L it is started at 30 mg.

- The treatment is continued for 18 months, as this appears to represent the length of therapy which is generally optimal in producing the remission rate of 40% at 5 years after discontinuing therapy.

- Relapses are most likely to occur within the first year and may be more likely in the presence of a large goitre and high T_3 level at the time of diagnosis.

Block and replace regime

- After achieving an euthyroid state on carbimazole alone, carbimazole at a dose of 40 mg daily together with T_4 at a dose of 100 µg can be prescribed. This is usually continued for 6 months.

- The main advantages are fewer hospital visits for checks of thyroid function and shorter duration of treatment.

- The originally reported higher remission rate was not confirmed in a large prospective multicentre European trial when combination treatment was compared to carbimazole alone.

- Relapses are most likely to occur within the first year and may be more likely in the presence of a large goitre and high T_3 level at the time of diagnosis.

- Much more common are the allergic type reactions of fever, rash, urticaria, and arthralgia, which occur in 1–5% of patients taking these drugs. These side-effects are often mild and do not usually necessitate drug withdrawal, although one ATD may be substituted for another in the expectation that the second agent may be taken without side-effects.

- Agranulocytosis represents a serious but rare side-effect of ATD occurring in 0.1–0.5% of patients. It occurs with equal frequency with carbimazole and propylthiouracil and because cross reactivity of this reaction has been reported, one drug should never be substituted for the other after this reaction has been diagnosed. Agranulocytosis usually occurs within the first 3 months after initiation of therapy but it is important to be aware of the documented cases, which have occurred (less frequently) a long time after starting treatment.

- As agranulocytosis occurs very suddenly, routine monitoring of full blood count is thought to be of little use. Patients typically present with fever and evidence of infection, usually in the oropharynx, and **each patient should therefore receive written instructions to discontinue the medication and contact their doctor for a blood count should the situation arise.**

Radioiodine therapy

Indications

- definitive treatment of multinodular goitre or adenoma
- relapsed Graves' disease.

Contra-indications

- young children, because of the potential risk of thyroid carcinogenesis.

- pregnant and lactating women.

- situations where it is clear that the safety of other people cannot be guaranteed

- *Graves' ophthalmopathy.* There is some evidence that Graves' ophthalmopathy may worsen after the administration of radioactive iodine, especially in smokers. In cases of moderate to severe ophthalmopathy radioiodine may be avoided. Alternatively steroid cover in a dose of 40 mg prednisolone should be administered on the day of administering radioiodine, 30 mg daily for the next 2 weeks, 20 mg daily for the following 2 weeks, reducing to zero over subsequent 3 weeks.

Radioiodine treatment

Clinical guidelines

The recommendation is to administer enough radioiodine to achieve euthyroidism with the acceptance of a moderate rate of hypothyroidism, e.g. 15–20% at 2 years and 1–3% per annum thereafter.

Instructions to patients

* Discontinue ATDs 2 days before radioiodine administration since their effects last for 24 h or more, though propylthiouracil has a prolonged radioprotective effect. ATDs may be recommenced 3 days or more after radioiodine administration without significantly affecting the delivered radiation dose.
* Patients should not have close contact (<1 m) with children under the age of 11 years for about 2 weeks after treatment.

Administration of radioiodine

* Radioactive iodine-131 is administered orally as a capsule or a drink.
* There is no universal agreement regarding the optimal dose. Dosing according to size alone is not successful in 90% of cases.
* A dose of 400–800 MBq should be sufficient to cure thyrotoxicosis in 90%. This would also render 50% of patients hypothyroid within 10 years.

Outcomes of radioiodine treatment

* In general 50–70% of patients have restored normal thyroid function and shrinkage of goitre within 6–8 weeks of receiving radioiodine.
* Persistent hyperthyroidism is treated by a further one or two administrations, at least 6 months apart.

(Reference: *The use of radioiodine in the management of hyperthyroidism.* Royal College of Physicians of London, November 1995)

Caveats

- The control of disease may not occur for a period of weeks or a few months.

- More than one treatment may be needed in some patients, depending on the dose given; 15% require a second dose and a few patients require a third dose. The second dose should be considered only at least 6 months after the first dose.

- Compounds that contain iodine, such as amiodarone, block iodine uptake for a period of several months following cessation of therapy; iodine uptake measurements may be helpful in this instance in determining the activity required and the timing of radioiodine therapy.

- Women of childbearing age should avoid pregnancy for a minimum of 4 months following radioactive iodine ablation.

- The incidence of hypothyroidism is about 50% at 10 years, and continues to occur thereafter.

Side-effects

- nausea and anterior neck pain caused by radiation-induced thyroiditis

- transient rise in thyroid hormone levels which may exacerbate heart failure if present.

Hypothyroidism after radioiodine

- After radioiodine administration, ATDs may be recommenced. The ATDs should be withdrawn gradually guided by a 6–8 weekly thyroid function test. Early post-radioiodine hypothyroidism may be transient. TSH should be monitored every 6 months after radioiodine to determine late hypothyroidism.

- In patients treated for autonomous toxic nodules the incidence of hypothyroidism is much lower since the toxic nodule takes up the radioactive iodine while the surrounding tissue will recover normal function once the hyperthyroidism is controlled, though this is disputed by some experts.

Cancer risk after radioiodine therapy

- In a recent large series, no overall excess risk of cancer was found. It is unclear whether the risk of thyroid cancer is slightly increased.

Table 3.3 Recommended activity of radioiodine

Aetiology	Comments	Guide dose (MBq)
Graves' disease	First presentation; no significant eye disease Moderate goitre (40–50 g)	400–550
Toxic multinodular goitre in older person	Mild heart failure; atrial fibrillation or other concomitant disease, e.g. cancer	At least 550
Toxic adenoma	Usually mild hyperthyroidism	300–500
Severe Graves' disease with thyroid eye disease	Postpone radioiodine till eye disease stable. Prednisolone 40 mg to be administered at same time as radioiodine and for further 4–6 weeks (p. 29)	400–550
Ablation therapy	Severe accompanying medical condition such as heart failure; atrial fibrillation or other concurrent medical disorders (e.g. psychosis)	800

Reference: *The use of radioiodine in the management of hyperthyroidism.* Royal College of Physicians of London, November 1995.

Surgery

Indications

- Documented suspicious or malignant thyroid nodule by FNAC.
- Pregnant mothers who are not adequately controlled by ATDs or in whom serious allergic reactions develop while being treated medically. Thyroidectomy is usually performed in the second trimester.
- Patients:
  - who reject or fear exposure to radiation
  - with poor compliance to medical treatment
  - in whom a rapid control of symptoms is desired
  - with severe manifestations of Graves' ophthalmopathy, as total or near total thyroidectomy does not worsen eye manifestations
  - with relapsed Graves' disease.
  - with local compressive symptoms which may not improve rapidly with radioiodine, whereas operation removes these symptoms in most patients
  - with large thyroid glands and relatively low radioiodine uptake.

Preparation of patients for surgery

- ATDs should be used preoperatively to achieve euthyroidism.
- Propranolol may be added to achieve ß-blockade especially in those patients where surgery must be performed sooner than achieving euthyroid state.
- Occasionally, potassium iodide, 60 mg 3xdaily can be used during the preoperative period to prevent an unwanted liberation of thyroid hormones during surgery. Preoperatively it should be given for 10 days. Operating later than this can be associated with exacerbation of thyrotoxicosis as the thyroid escapes from the inhibitory effect of the iodide. In practice it is rarely needed as good control of thyrotoxicosis can be achieved with ATDs in the majority of patients. Lugol's iodine should not be used because of its variable iodine content.

Hypothyroidism after surgery

- Reported incidence of hypothyroidism following subtotal thyroidectomy is around 10–20% at 10 years and continues to rise inexorably.
- A small remnant size(<4 g) results in a high incidence(>50%) of hypothyroidism
- Thyroid antibody activity and infiltration of the gland by lymphocytes cause destruction of the gland and hypothyroidism.

- If the thyroid remnant is 8 g or larger, there is an increase in the incidence of persistent or recurrent disease (approximately 15%).
- The best centres achieve less than 4% recurrence. Cure (i.e. low recurrence) inevitably means a high rate of long-term hypothyroidism.

Table 3.4 Complications of thyroidectomy

Immediate	Late
Recurrent laryngeal nerve damage	Hypothyroidism
Hypoparathyroidism	Keloid formation
Thyroid crisis	
Local haemorrhage, causing laryngeal oedema	
Wound infection	

Thyroid storm (crisis)

Thyroid crisis represents a rare but life threatening exacerbation of the manifestations of thyrotoxicosis. It should be promptly recognized since the condition is associated with a significant mortality (30–50% depending on series). Thyroid crisis develops in hyperthyroid patients who

- have an acute infection
- undergo thyroidal or non thyroidal surgery or radioiodine treatment
- are postpartum
- receive radiographic contrast agents
- have had ATDs withdrawn.

Thyroid crisis should be considered in a very sick patient if there is:

- recent past history suggestive of thyrotoxicosis
- acute stressful precipitating factor such as surgery
- history of previous thyroid treatment
- family history of a thyroid disorder.

Treatment

General supportive therapy

- The patient is best managed in an intensive care unit where close attention can be paid to the cardiorespiratory status, fluid balance, and cooling.
- Standard anti-arrhythmic drugs can be used, including digoxin (usually in higher than normal dose) after correction for hypokalaemia. If anticoagulation is indicated because of atrial fibrillation then it must be remembered that thyrotoxic patients are very sensitive to warfarin.
- Chlorpromazine (50–100 mg i/m) can be used to treat agitation and because of its effect in inhibiting central thermoregulation it may be useful in treating the hyperpyrexia.
- Broad-spectrum antibiotics should be given if infection is suspected.

Specific treatment

- Aim: to inhibit thyroid hormone synthesis completely.
- Propylthiouracil 200–300 mg 6 hourly via nasogastric tube. Propylthiouracil is preferred because of its ability to block T_4 to T_3 conver-

Thyroid storm

Clinical signs suggestive of a thyroid storm

- alteration in mental status
- high fever
- tachycardia or tachyarrhythmias
- severe clinical hyperthyroid signs
- vomiting, jaundice, and diarrhoea
- multisystem decompensation: cardiac failure, respiratory distress, congestive hepatomegaly, dehydration, and prerenal failure.

Laboratory investigation

- Routine haematology may indicate a leukocytosis, which is well-recognized in thyrotoxicosis even in the absence of infection.
- The biochemical screen may reveal a raised alkaline phosphatase and mild hypercalcaemia.
- Thyroid function tests and thyroid antibodies should be requested although treatment should not be delayed while awaiting the results
- The levels of thyroid hormones will be raised but may not be grossly elevated and are usually within the range of uncomplicated thyrotoxicosis

sion in peripheral tissues. There are no clinical data comparing propylthiouracil and carbimazole in this situation

- Potassium iodide 60 mg via nasogastric tube, 6 hourly, 6 h *after* starting propylthiouracil will inhibit thyroid hormone release.
- β-Adrenergic blocking agents are essential in the management to control tachycardia, tremor, and other adrenergic manifestations: Propranolol 160–480 mg/day in divided doses or as an infusion at a rate of 2–5 mg/h.
- Calcium channel blockers can be tried in patients with known bronchospastic disease where ß-blockade is contraindicated.
- High doses of glucocorticoids may help to stabilize the vascular bed and are capable of blocking T_4 to T_3 conversion: Prednisolone 60 mg daily or hydrocortisone 40 mg i/m, 4× daily.
- Plasmapheresis and peritoneal dialysis may be effective in cases resistant to the usual pharmacological measures.

Subclinical hyperthyroidism

* Subclinical hyperthyroidism is defined as undetectable thyrotropin (TSH) concentration in patients with normal levels of T_4 and T_3. Subtle symptoms and signs of thyrotoxicosis may be present.

* May be classified as endogenous in patients with thyroid hormone production associated with nodular thyroid disease or underlying Graves' disease; and as exogenous in those with undetectable serum thyrotropin concentrations as a result of treatment with levothyroxine.

* The evidence that subclinical hyperthyroidism is a risk factor for the development of atrial fibrillation or osteoporosis is not definitive.

  * There is only limited evidence that established atrial fibrillation in patients with subclinical hyperthyroidism reverts spontaneously or after cardioversion once the serum thyrotropin concentration has been normalized with antithyroid therapy. Available evidence suggest that among patients with atrial fibrillation that is unrelated to rheumatic heart disease, those with thyrotoxicosis have a higher rate of embolism than do patients without the condition.

  * The increased risk of fracture reported in older women taking thyroid hormone disappears when those with a history of hyperthyroidism are excluded.

* The natural history of subclinical hyperthyroidism remains unclear. In statements issued in 1996 and 1998 respectively, the Royal College of Physicians of London and the American College of Physicians concluded that there is no agreement about the benefits of detecting and treating endogenous subclinical hyperthyroidism or about whether it causes excess morbidity. However an expert panel of the American Thyroid Association has recommended routine screening of adults for thyroid disease by measurement of serum thyrotropin.

* In many patients with endogeneous subclinical hyperthyroidism who do not have nodular thyroid disease or complications of excess thyroid hormone, treatment is unnecessary, but thyroid-function tests should be performed every six months. In older patients with atrial fibrillation or osteoporosis that could have been caused or exacerbated by the mild excess of thyroid hormone, ablative therapy with ^{131}I is the best initial option.

- In patients with exogeneous subclinical hyperthyroidism, the dose of thyroxine should be reduced, excluding those with prior thyroid cancer in whom thyrotropin suppression may be required. Dose of thyroxine used for treating hypothyroidism may be reduced if the patient develops
  - new atrial fibrillation, angina or cardiac failure
  - accelerated bone loss
  - borderline high serum triiodothyronine concentration

Thyrotoxic hypokalaemic periodic paralysis

- Thyrotoxic
- Potassium loss
- Intermittent muscle weakness + CPK ↑
- Precipitated by heavy exertion or CHO load
- More common in Asians

Thyrotoxicosis in pregnancy (See p. 501)

* Thyrotoxicosis occurs in about 0.2% of pregnancies
* Graves' disease accounts for 90% of cases
* Less common causes include toxic adenoma and multinodular goitre
* Other causes are hyperemesis gravidarum and trophoblastic neoplasia

Diagnosis of thyrotoxicosis during pregnancy may be difficult or delayed.

* Physiological changes of pregnancy are similar to those of hyperthyroidism.
* Total T_4 and T_3 are elevated in pregnancy because of an elevated level of TBG but, with free hormone assays available, this is no longer a problem.
* Physiological features of normal pregnancy include an increase in basal metabolic rate, cardiac stroke volume, palpitations, and heat intolerance.
* Serum free T_3 concentrations remain within the normal range in most pregnant women; serum TSH concentration decreases during the first trimester.

Symptoms

* Hyperemesis gravidarum is the classic presentation. Tiredness, palpitations, insomnia, heat intolerance, proximal muscle weakness, shortness of breath, and irritability may be other presenting symptoms.
* Thyrotoxicosis may occasionally be diagnosed when the patient presents with pregnancy-induced hypertension or congestive heart failure.

Signs

* failure to gain weight despite a good appetite
* persistent tachycardia with a pulse rate >90 beats/min at rest
* other signs of thyrotoxicosis as described previously

Natural history of Graves' disease in pregnancy

* There is aggravation of symptoms in the first half of the pregnancy; amelioration of symptoms in the second half of the pregnancy, and often recurrence of symptoms in the postpartum period.

Transient hyperthyroidism of hyperemesis gravidarum

- The likely mechanism is a raised β-hCG level.
- βHCG, LH, FSH, and TSH are glycoprotein hormones that contain a common α-subunit and a hormone-specific β-subunit. There is an inverse relationship between the serum levels of TSH and hCG, best seen in early pregnancy. There is also structural homology of the TSH and hCG receptors.
- Serum free T_4 concentration may be increased and the TSH levels suppressed in women with hyperemesis gravidarum.
- Thyroid function tests recover after the resolution of hyperemesis.
- Pregnant women with hyperemesis gravidarum should not be given ATD treatment but managed supportively with fluids, antiemetics, and nutritional support.
- There is no increased risk of thyrotoxicosis in subsequent pregnancies.
- Can be differentiated from Graves' disease by the presence of antithyroid antibodies, or family history of Graves' disease, a history of other autoimmune phenomena and a previous history of ophthalmic Graves'
- The dosage of ATDs is frequently adjusted during the course of the pregnancy; therefore thyroid tests should be done at 2–4 week intervals, with the goal of keeping free thyroid hormone levels in the upper one-third of the reference range.

Management of Graves' disease in the mother

- Aim of treatment is alleviation of thyroid symptoms and normalization of tests in the shortest time. Patients should be seen every 4–8 weeks and TFTs performed. Serum free T_4 is the best test to follow the response to ATDs. Block and replace regime should not be used as this will result in fetal hypothyroidism.

- Both PTU (150 mg b.d.) and carbimazole (10–20 mg once daily) are effective in controlling the disease in pregnancy. As propylthiouracil is more bound to plasma proteins, theoretically less drug would be transferred to the foetus. Compliance with carbimazole might be better. A β-blocker (propranolol 20–40 mg 6–8 hourly) is effective in controlling the hypermetabolic symptoms but should be used only for a few weeks until symptoms abate.

- Thyroid tests may normalize spontaneously with the progression of a normal pregnancy as a result of immunological changes.

- The use of iodides and radioiodine is contraindicated in pregnancy.

- Surgery is rarely performed in pregnancy. It is reserved for patients not responding to ATDs. It is preferable to perform surgery in the second trimester.

- Breast-feeding mothers should be treated with the lowest possible dose of propylthiouracil.

Prepregnancy counselling

- Hyperthyroid women who want to conceive should attain euthyroidism before conception, as stillbirth due to cranial synostosis is the most serious complication.

- There is no evidence that radioactive iodine treatment given to the mother 4 months or more before pregnancy has an adverse effect on the foetus or on an offspring in later life.

- Antithyroid medication requirements decrease during gestation; in about 50–60% of women the dose may be discontinued in the last few weeks of gestation.

- The risk of postpartum thyroiditis or recurrent hyperthyroidism should be discussed with the patient

- The rare occurrence of foetal and neonatal hyperthyroidism should be included during counselling sessions.

Management of the foetus

* The hypothalamopituitary thyroid axis is well developed at 12 weeks gestation but remains inactive until 18–20 weeks. Circulating TSH receptor antibodies (TSH-RAB) in the mother can cross the placenta. The risk of hyperthyroidism to the neonate can be assessed by measuring TSH-RAB in the maternal circulation at the beginning of the third trimester. Antithyroglobulin antibody and thyroid peroxidase antibodies have no effect on the foetus.

* Long-term follow-up studies of children whose mothers received either carbimazole or propylthiouracil have not shown an increased incidence of any physical or psychological defects. The block and replace regime using relatively high doses of carbimazole is contra-indicated because the ATDs cross the placenta, but replacement T_4 does not, thus potentially rendering the foetus hypothyroid.

* Monitoring the foetal heart rate and growth rates are the standard means whereby foetal thyrotoxicosis may be detected. A rate above 160 beats/min is suspicious of foetal thyrotoxicosis in the third trimester. Foetal thyrotoxicosis may complicate the latter part of the pregnancy of women with Graves' disease even if they have previously been treated with radioiodine or surgery. If there is evidence of foetal thyrotoxicosis, the dose of the ATD should be increased. If this causes maternal hypothyroidism a small dose of T_4 can be added since, unlike carbimazole, T_4 does not cross the placenta. A paediatrician should be involved to monitor neonatal thyroid function and detect thyrotoxicosis.

* Hypothyroidism in the mother should be avoided because of the potential adverse effect on subsequent cognitive function of the neonate.

* If the mother has been treated with carbimazole, the post-delivery levels of T_4 may be low and neonatal levels of T_4 may only rise to the thyrotoxic range after a few days. In addition, TSH is usually absent in neonates who subsequently develop thyrotoxicosis. Clinical indicators of neonatal thyrotoxicosis include low birth weight, poor weight gain, tachycardia, and irritability. Carbimazole can be given at a dose of 0.5 mg/kg per day and withdrawn after a few weeks after the level of TSH-RAB declines.

Thyrotoxicosis presenting in the postpartum period

- Defined as a syndrome of postpartum thyrotoxicosis or hypothyroidism in women who were euthyroid during pregnancy.

- Postpartum thyroid dysfunction, which occurs in women with autoimmune thyroid disease, is characterized in a third by a thyrotoxic phase occurring in the first 3 months postpartum, followed by a hypothyroid phase that occurs 3–6 months after delivery, followed by spontaneous recovery. In the remaining two-thirds, single-phase pattern or the reverse occurs.

- 5–7 % percent of women develop biochemical evidence of thyroid dysfunction after delivery. An increased risk is seen in patients with type I diabetes mellitus (25%), other autoimmune diseases, in the presence of anti-TPO antibodies and in the presence of a family history of thyroid disease.

- Hyperthyroidism due to Graves' disease accounts for 10–15% of all cases of postpartum thyrotoxicosis. In the majority of cases, hyperthyroidism occurs later in the postpartum period (>3–6 months) and persists.

- Providing the patient is not breast-feeding, a radioiodine uptake scan can differentiate the two principal causes of autoimmune thyrotoxicosis by demonstrating increased uptake in Graves' disease and low uptake in postpartum thyroiditis. In fact, ^{99m}Tc can be usefully employed in breast-feeding which need be discontinued for 24 h only.

- Graves' hyperthyroidism should be treated with ATDs. Propylthiouracil is preferable if the patient is breast-feeding. Thyrotoxic symptoms due to postpartum thyrotoxicosis are managed symptomatically using propranolol.

- One-third of affected women develop symptoms of hypothyroidism and may require T_4 for 6–12 months. There is a suggestion of an increased risk of postpartum depression in those with hypothyroidism.

- Histology of the thyroid in the case of postpartum thyroiditis shows lymphocytic infiltration with destructive thyroiditis and predominantly occurs at 16 weeks in women with positive antimicrosomal antibodies.

- There is an increased chance of subsequent permanent hypothyroidism in 25–30%. Patients should be followed up with annual TSH measurements.

Table 3.6 Potential maternal and foetal complications in uncontrolled hyperthyroidism in pregnancy

Maternal	Foetal
Pregnancy induced hypertension	Hyperthyroidism
Preterm delivery	Neonatal hyperthyroidism
Congestive heart failure	Intrauterine growth retardation
Thyroid storm	Small-for-gestation age
Miscarriage	Prematurity
Abruptio placentae	Stillbirth: cranial synostosis is the most serious complication

Hyperthyroidism in children

Epidemiology

Thyrotoxicosis is rare before the age of 5 years. Although there is a progressive increase in incidence throughout childhood it is still rare and accounts for less than 5% of all cases of Graves' disease.

Clinical features

• Behavioural abnormalities, hyperactivity, declining school performance may bring the child to medical attention. Features of hyperthyroidism as described previously.

• Acceleration of linear growth is common in patients increasing in height percentiles on the growth charts. The disease may be part of McCune–Albright syndrome and café-au-lait pigmentation, precocious puberty, and bony abnormalities should be considered during clinical examination.

Investigations

The cause of thyrotoxicosis in children is nearly always Graves' disease (with positive antibodies to thyroglobulin, thyroid peroxidase, or both) although thyroiditis and toxic nodules have been described and a radioiodine scan may be useful if the diagnosis is not clear. Hereditary thyroid-resistant syndromes often misdiagnosed as Graves' disease are now being increasingly recognized in children.

Treatment

ATDs represent the treatment of choice for thyrotoxic children. Therapy is generally started with Propylthiouracil 2–4 mg/kg (Initial dose 100–150 mg/day) or carbimazole 0.2–0.4 mg/kg (initial dose 10–15 mg/day).

Secondary hyperthyroidism

- Thyrotoxicosis resulting from primary TSH overproduction by the pituitary gland with secondary thyroid enlargement and hyperfunction.

- Causes:
  - TSH-producing pituitary tumours (TSHomas)
  - syndrome of resistance to thyroid hormones.

- There are characteristically *elevated* serum free T_4 and T_3 concentrations and *non-suppressed* (inappropriately normal or frankly elevated) serum TSH levels.

- Among the 280 TSHomas reported in the literature (till 1998), 72% secreted TSH alone; the remainder co-secreted growth hormone (16%), prolactin (11%), or rarely gonadotrophins. Approximately 90% were macroadenomas (>1 cm in diameter) and 71% exhibited suprasellar extension, invasion, or both into adjacent tissues (see p. 219).

- Patients with pure TSHomas present with typical symptoms and signs of thyrotoxicosis and the presence of a diffuse goitre. Unilateral exophthalmos from tumour invasion of the orbit and bilateral exophthalmos have been reported. Patients may exhibit features of over secretion of the other pituitary hormones, e.g. prolactin or growth hormone. Headaches, visual field defects, menstrual irregularities, amenorrhoea, delayed puberty, and hypogonadotrophic hypogonadism have also been reported. Careful establishment of the diagnosis is the key to treatment. Inappropriate treatment of such patients with subtotal thyroidectomy or radioiodine administration not only fails to cure the underlying disorder but also seems to be associated with subsequent pituitary tumour enlargement and an increased risk of invasiveness into adjacent tissues.

- Treatment options are
  - transphenoidal surgery
  - pituitary radiotherapy if surgical results are unsatisfactory, or surgery is contraindicated or not desired
  - medical therapy with somatostatin analogues such as octreotide or lanreotide may be useful preoperatively and suppresses TSH secretion in 80% of the cases.

Resistance to thyroid hormones

* Patients with generalized resistance to thyroid hormone (GRTH) may present with mild hypothyroidism, deaf mutism, delayed bone maturation, raised circulating thyroid hormone concentrations, non-suppressed TSH, and failure of TSH to decrease normally upon administration of supraphysiological doses of thyroid hormones. Most patients present with goitre or incidentally abnormal TFTs. Treatment is determined by thyroid status.

* In selective pituitary resistance to thyroid hormones (PRTH) the thyroid hormone resistance is more pronounced in the pituitary; thus the patient exhibits definite clinical manifestations of thyrotoxicosis.

* About 90% of thyroid hormone resistance syndromes result from mutations in the gene encoding *TR β*. Mutant receptors have a reduced affinity for T_3 and are functionally deficient. It is usually inherited in an autosomal dominant pattern with the affected individuals being heterozygous for the mutation.

* A subset of RTH receptors has been identified that are capable of inhibiting wild type receptor action. When co-expressed, the mutant proteins are able to inhibit the function of their wild type counterparts in a dominant negative manner.

* Common features of patients with the thyroid hormones resistance syndromes include goitre, tachycardia, hyperkinetic behaviour, emotional disturbances, ear nose and throat infections, language disabilities, auditory disorders, low body weight, cardiac abnormalities, and subnormal intelligence quotients.

* Treatment options after carefully establishing the diagnosis in PRTH include:

  - Chronic suppression of TSH secretion with D T4, triiodothyroacetic acid, octreotide, or bromocriptine
  - If above ineffective, thyroid ablation with radioiodine or surgery with subsequent close monitoring of thyroid hormone status and pituitary gland size.

Table 3.5 Tests useful in the differential diagnosis of TSHomas, PRTH, and GRTH

Test	TSHomas	PRTH	GRTH
Clinical thyrotoxicosis	Present	Present	Absent
Family history	Absent	Present	Present
TSH response to TRH	No change	Increase	Increase
TSH response to low dose T_3	No change	Decrease	Decrease
SHBG	Elevated[a]	Normal[b]	Normal
Pituitary MRI	Tumour[c]	Normal	Normal

[a] Not raised in mixed GH/TSH tumour.

[b] Peripheral markers of toxicosis sometimes affected.

[c] The best biochemical test is α-subunit

Chapter 4
Graves' ophthalmopathy, dermopathy, and acropachy

Graves' ophthalmopathy

- An organ-specific autoimmune disorder characterized by swelling of the extra-ocular muscles, lymphocytic infiltration, late fibrosis, muscle tethering, and proliferation of orbital fat and connective tissue.

- There are two stages in the development of the disease, which can be recognized as an active inflammatory (dynamic) stage and a relatively quiescent static stage. 5% of patients with Graves' ophthalmopathy have hypothyroidism and 5% are euthyroid. 75% of patients develop Graves' disease within a year either side of Graves' ophthalmopathy developing. The lesions are due to localized accumulation of glycosaminoglycans.

- The appearance of eye disease follows a different time course to thyroid dysfunction and in a minority there is a lag period between the presentation of hyperthyroidism and the appearance of eye signs.

- Smoking and hypothyroidism moderately worsen Graves' ophthalmopathy.

- The role of an endocrinologist during a routine review of Graves' patients is to record accurately the clinical features of Graves' eye disease and to identify ocular emergencies, such as corneal ulceration, congestive ophthalmopathy, and optic neuropathy, which should be referred urgently to an ophthalmologist.

Clinical features

- Retraction of eyelids is extremely common in thyroid eye disease. The margin of the upper eyelid normally rests about 2 mm below the limbus and retraction can be suspected if the lid margin is either level or above the superior limbus allowing the sclera to be visible. The lower lid normally rests at the inferior limbus and retraction is suspected when the sclera shows above the lid.

- Proptosis can result in failure of lid closure, increasing the likelihood of exposure keratitis and the common symptom of gritty eyes. This can be confirmed with a fluorescein or Rose Bengal stain. As papilloedema can occur, fundoscopy should be performed. Proptosis may result in periorbital oedema and chemosis because the displaced orbit results in less efficient lachrymal drainage.

- Persistent visual blurring may indicate an optic neuropathy and requires urgent treatment.

- Severe conjunctival pain may indicate corneal ulceration requiring urgent referral.

Investigation of proptosis

- *Documentation using a Hertel exophthalmometer* The feet of the apparatus are placed against the lateral orbital margin as defined by the zygomatic bones. The marker on the body of the exophthalmometer is then superimposed on the reflection of the contralateral one by adjusting the scale. The position of each cornea can be read off against the reflections on a milli-metre scale as seen on the mirror of the apparatus. A normal result is generally taken as being <20 mm. A reading of 21 mm or more is abnormal and a difference of 2 mm between the eyes is suspicious.

- *Soft tissue involvement* Soft tissue signs and symptoms include conjunctival hyperaemia, chemosis, tearing, and foreign body sensation. The soft tissue changes can be secondary to exposure and lagophthalmos but are often seen in the absence of these aetiological factors.

- *CT or MRI scan of the orbit* demonstrates enlargement of the extra-ocular muscles and this can be useful in cases of diagnostic difficulty. This is also more accurate for demonstration of proptosis.

Table 4.1 Treatment of Graves' ophthalmopathy

Problem	Treatment
Grittiness	Artificial tears and simple eye ointment
Eyelid retraction	Tape eyelids at night to avoid corneal damage. Surgery if risk of exposure keratopathy
Proptosis	Head elevation during sleep Diuretics Systemic steroids Radiotherapy Orbital decompression
Optic neuropathy	Systemic steroids Radiotherapy Orbital decompression
Ophthalmoplegia	Prisms in the acute phase Orbital decompression Orbital muscle surgery

Examining for possible optic neuropathy

- History of *poor vision*, a recent or *rapid change in vision*, or *poor colour vision* are reasons for prompt referral.

- *A visual acuity* of less than 6/18 warrants referral to an ophthalmologist. For *colour vision*, each eye should be evaluated by using a simple 15-plate Ishihara colour vision test. Decreased colour vision is a subtle indicator of optic nerve function. Failure to identify more than 2 of the plates with either eye is an indication for referral. This is unhelpful in the 8% of men who may be colour blind.

- *Marcus Gunn pupil* The 'swinging flashlight' test detects the presence of an *afferent pupillary defect*.

Ophthalmoplegia

- Patients may complain of diplopia due to ocular muscle dysfunction caused by either oedema during the early active phase or fibrosis during the later phase. Assessment using a Hess chart may be helpful. Intra-optic pressure may increase on upgaze and result in compression of the globe by a fibrotic inferior rectus muscle. Ocular mobility may be restricted by oedema during the active inflammatory phase or by fibrosis during the fibrotic stage.

- The two most common findings are defective elevation caused by fibrotic contraction of the inferior rectus muscle and a convergence defect caused by fibrotic contraction of the medial rectus. Disorders of the medial rectus, superior rectus, and lateral rectus muscle produce typical signs of defective adduction, depression and abduction respectively.

Treatment

Eyelid retraction

- Most patients do not require any treatment, since clinical signs usually improve with treatment of hyperthyroidism or spontaneously with time (27%). In patients with significant lid retraction and exposure keratopathy, surgery to reduce the vertical lid fissures can be considered.

- Orbital decompression and strabismus surgery, if required, should be considered before eyelid surgery because the outcome of these influences the eyelid position.

- Surgery to correct lid-lag retraction, soft tissue abnormalities including periorbital laxity, and ophthalmoplegia, may be performed once the active phase has resolved and the patient is euthyroid

Graves' dermopathy

- This is a rare complication of Graves' thyrotoxicosis. It is usually pre-tibial in location and hence called *pre-tibial myxoedema*.
- It typically appears as raised, discoloured, and indurated lesions on the front or back of the legs, or on the dorsum of the feet, and has occasionally been described in other areas, including the hands and the face.
- The lesions are due to localized accumulation of *glycosamino-glycans*. It is now recognized that there is a lymphocytic infiltrate. Lesions are characteristically asymptomatic but they can also be pruritic and tender. They can be very disfiguring.
- *Treatment* Usually not treated. Potent topical fluorinated steroids such as fluocinolone acetonide are effective, not only in the treatment of localized pain and tenderness but also in some resolution of the visible skin signs. Severe pre-tibial myxo-edema may require systemic steroids in conjunction with compression bandages. Surgery may worsen the condition.

Thyroid acropachy

- This is the rarest manifestation of Graves' disease.
- It presents as clubbing of the digits and sub-periosteal new bone formation. The soft tissue swelling is similar to that seen in localized myxoedema and consists of glycosaminoglycan accumulation.
- Patients almost inevitably have Graves' ophthalmopathy or pretibial myxoedema. If not, an alternative cause of clubbing should be looked for.
- It is typically painless and there is no effective treatment.

Soft tissue involvement

- Artificial tears and liquid paraffin eye ointment (Lacri-Lube) may give symptom relief. Head elevation during sleep or diuretics may reduce morning orbital oedema.

Proptosis

- Severe proptosis prevents adequate lid closure and may lead to exposure keratopathy and corneal ulceration. Systemic steroids, orbital radiotherapy. or surgery may be considered in those patients with very active disease. Intravenous methyl prednisolone, 500 mg daily, repeated on three consecutive days may produce a rapid response, which can be continued with a course of oral prednisolone. Oral prednisolone can be tried from the outset although high doses of at least 60 mg daily are usually required and adverse affects may be a disadvantage. The dose of prednisolone should be reduced over the subsequent few weeks, depending on the clinical response.

- Orbital radiotherapy may also be considered early in the course of active inflammatory eye disease.

- Orbital surgical decompression.

Optic neuropathy

- Oral corticosteroids, orbital decompression, and radiotherapy have been used extensively.

- Oral prednisolone, 80 mg/day, in divided doses should be given for 2 weeks and then tapered gradually to zero. Lack of improvement or recurrence should prompt surgical intervention.

- Orbital decompression surgery aims to release pressure on the optic nerve in the posterior orbit where the muscles are tremendously enlarged. The medial wall or lamina papyracea and orbital floor are removed.

- Radiotherapy works slowly and is usually a method of last resort. Corticosteroids are given at the same time to avoid the initial worsening of symptoms. Complications include radiation keratitis and retinitis, which occur rarely.

Ophthalmoplegia

- Temporary measures such as occluding one eyeglass lens, or the use of a Fresnel prism on one or both lenses, are beneficial.

- Complex surgery on several ocular muscles is often indicated. Multiple operations may be necessary.

Further reading

Brix TH, Kyvik KO, Hegedus L. What is the evidence of genetic factors in the etiology of Graves' disease? A brief review. *Thyroid* 1998; 8: 727–34.

Fatourechi V, Pajouhi M, Fransway AF. Dermopathy of Graves disease (pretibial myxedema). Review of 150 cases. *Medicine* (Baltimore) 1994; 73: 1–7.

Franklyn JA. The management of hyperthyroidism *N Engl J Med* 1994; 330: 1731–1738 [Erratum *N Engl J Med* 1994; 331:559].

Franklyn JA, Maisonneuve P, Sheppard MC, Betteridge J, Boyle P. Mortality after the treatment of hyperthyroidism with radioactive iodine *N Engl J Med* 1998; 338: 172–718.

Franklyn JA, Maisonneuve P, Sheppard MC, Betteridge J, Boyle P. Cancer incidence and mortality after radioiodine treatment for hyperthyroidism: a population-based cohort study *Lancet* 1999; 353: 2111–2115.

Gunji K, Kubota S, Swanson J *et al.* Role of the eye muscles in thyroid eye disease: identification of the principal autoantigens. *Thyroid* 1998; 8:553–556 [Erratum *Thyroid* 1998; 8: 1079].

Heufelder AE. Pathogenesis of Graves' ophthalmopathy: recent controversies and progress *Eur J of Endocrinol* 1995; 132: 532–541.

Heward JM, Allahabadis A, Daykin J *et al.* Linkage disequilibrium between the human leukocyte antigen class II region of the major histocompatibility complex and Graves' disease: replication using a population case control and family-based study. *J of Clin Endocrinol Metab* 1998; 83: 3394–3397.

Laurberg P, Nygaard B, Glinoer D *et al.* Guidelines for TSH-receptor antibody measurements in pregnancy: results of an evidence-based symposium organized by the European Thyroid Association. *Eur J Endocrinol* 1998;139: 584–586.

Lazarus JH, Hall R, Ottman S, Barks AB *et al.* The clinical spectrum of postpartum thyroid disease *QJM* 1996; 89: 429–435.

Mandel SJ, Brent GA, Larsen PR. Review of antithyroid drug use during pregnancy and report of a case of aplasia cutis. *Thyroid* 1994; 4:129–133.

Mestman JH. Hyperthyroidism in pregnancy. *Endocrinol Metab Clin N America* 1998; 27(1): 127–149.

Perros P, Crombie AL, Matthews JNS, Kendall-Taylor P. Age and gender influence the severity of thyroid-associated ophthalmopathy: a study of 101 patients attending a combined thyroid-eye clinic. *Clin Endocrinol* (Oxf)1993; 38: 367–372.

Risk of agranulocytosis and aplastic anaemia in relation to use of antithyroid drugs. International Agranulocytosis and Aplastic Anaemia Study. *BMJ* 1988; 297: 262–265.

Rivkees SA, Sklar C, Freemark M. The management of Graves's disease in children, with special emphasis on radioiodine treatment. *J Clin Endocrinol Metab* 1998; 83: 3767–3776.

Ron E, Doody MM, Becker DV *et al.* Cancer mortality following treatment for adult hyperthyroidism. Cooperative Thyrotoxicosis Therapy Follow-up Study Group. *JAMA* 1998; 280: 347–355.

Tellez M, Cooper J, Edmonds C. Graves' ophthalmopathy in relation to cigarette smoking and ethnic origin. *Clin Endocrinol* (Oxf) 1992; 36: 291–294.

Toft AD. Clinical practice. Subclinical hyperthyroidism *New Engl J Med* 2001; 345(7): 512–516.

Toft AD, Weetman AP. Screening for agranulocytosis in patients treated with antithyroid drugs. *Clin Endocrinol* (Oxf) 1998; 49: 271.

Wartofsky L, Sherman SI, Gopal J, Schlumberger M, Hay ID. The use of radioactive iodine in patients with papillary and follicular thyroid cancer. *J Clin Endocrinol Metab* 1998; 83: 4195 –4203.

Weetman AP. Graves's disease *N Engl J Med* 2000; 343(17): 1236–1248.

Weetman AP, Pickerill AP, Watson P, Chatterjee VK, Edwarda OM. Treatment of Graves' disease with the block-replace regimen of antithyroid drugs: the effect of treatment duration and immunogenetic susceptibility on relapse. *QJM* 1994; 87: 337–341.

Chapter 5
Multinodular goitre and solitary adenomas

Background

Nodular thyroid disease denotes the presence of single or multiple palpable or non-palpable nodules within the thyroid gland.

- Prevalence rates range from 5–50% depending on population studied and sensitivity of detection methods. Prevalence increases linearly with age, exposure to ionizing radiation and iodine deficiency.
- Clinically apparent thyroid nodules are evident in ~10% of the UK population.
- Incidence of thyroid nodules is about 4 times more in women.
- Thyroid nodules always raise the concern of cancer, but <5% are cancerous.

Clinical evaluation

- An asymptomatic thyroid mass may be discovered either by a clinician on routine neck palpation or by the patient during self-examination.
- History should concentrate on
  - an enlarging thyroid mass
  - a previous history of radiation, especially childhood head and neck irradiation
  - a family history of thyroid cancer
  - the development of hoarseness or dysphagia.
- Nodules are more likely to be malignant in patients <20 or >60 years.
- Thyroid nodules are more common in women but more likely to be malignant in men.
- Physical findings suggestive of malignancy include a firm or hard non-tender nodule; a recent history of enlargement, fixation to adjacent tissue, and the presence of regional lymphadenopathy.
- A hot nodule on a radioisotope scan makes malignancy less likely.

Table 5.1 Aetiology of thyroid nodules

Common causes	Uncommon causes
Colloid nodule	Granulomatous thyroiditis
Cyst	Infections
Lymphocytic thyroiditis	Malignancy
Benign neoplasms	Medullary
Hurthle cell	Anaplastic
Follicular	Metastatic
Malignancy	Lymphoma
Papillary	
Follicular	

Clinical features raising the suspicion of thyroid malignancy

- age (childhood or elderly)
- short history of enlarging nodule
- local symptoms including dysphagia, stridor, or hoarseness
- previous exposure to radiation
- positive family history of thyroid cancer or MEN syndrome
- Gardner's syndrome (familial large intestinal polyposis)
- familial polyposis coli
- Cowden's syndrome (autosomal dominantly inherited hamartoma syndrome)
- lymphadenopathy
- history of Hashimoto's disease (increased incidence of lymphoma)

Investigations

- fine needle aspiration cytology (see p. 13)
- TSH
- pulmonary function tests especially for a large goitre causing tracheal obstruction
- CT scan if there are concerns about retrosternal goitre.

Treatment

Toxic multinodular goitre or nodule

The patient should initially be rendered euthyroid with medical treatment.

ATDs

- ATD are effective in controlling the hyperthyroidism but are not curative. As the hot nodules are autonomous the condition will recur after stopping the drugs. Carbimazole is useful treatment to gain control of the disease in preparation for surgery or as long-term treatment in those patients unwilling to accept radioiodine or surgery.

Radioiodine

- This form of treatment is often considered as first choice for definitive treatment. ^{131}I is preferentially accumulated in hot follicles but not in normal thyroid tissue which, because of the thyrotoxic state, is non-functioning.
- Radioiodine treatment commonly induces a euthyroid state as the hot follicles are destroyed and the previously non-functioning follicles gradually resume normal function.

Surgery

- The aim of surgery is to remove as much of the nodular tissue as possible and if the goitre is large to relieve local symptoms. Postoperative follow-up should involve checks of thyroid function.
- Goitre recurrence, although rare, does occasionally occur.

Non-toxic multinodular goitre

Surgery

Is the preferred treatment for patients with:

- local compression symptoms
- cosmetic disfigurement
- solitary nodule with FNAC suspicious of malignancy.

Radioiodine

- Radioiodine may be particularly indicated in elderly patients in whom surgery is not appropriate. Up to 50% shrinkage of goitre mass has been reported in recent studies.

- Hypothyroidism following radioiodine is low but is still recognized and seems to be related to the degree of TSH suppression and reduction in radioiodine uptake by the extranodular tissue.

Medical treatment

- Use of T_4 to suppress TSH is associated with risk of cardiac arrhythmias and bone loss. T_4 is useful only if TSH is detectable. It is less useful in nodular goitre.

Aetiology of goitre

- autoimmune thyroid disease
- sporadic
- endemic (iodine deficiency, dietary origins)
- pregnancy
- drug-induced (ATDs, lithium, amiodarone)
- thyroiditis syndromes.

Pathology

Thyroid nodules may be described as *adenomas* if the follicular cell differentiation is enclosed within a capsule; *adenomatous* when the lesions are circumscribed but not encapsulated.

Further reading

Gharib H. Changing concepts in the diagnosis and management of thyroid nodules. *Endocrinology and Metabolism Clinics of North America* 1997; 26(4): 777–800.

Chapter 6
Thyroiditis

Background

Inflammation of the thyroid gland often leads to a transient thyrotoxicosis followed by hypothyroidism. Overt hypothyroidism caused by autoimmunity has two main forms: *Hashimoto's (goitrous) thyroiditis* and *atrophic thyroiditis (myxoedema)*

Table 6.1 Causes and characteristics of thyroiditis

Cause	Characteristic features
Pyogenic	*Staph. aureus*, streptococci, *E. coli*, tuberculosis, fungal
Sub-acute (de Quervain) (p. 67)	Thought to be viral in origin, multinuclear giant cells
Autoimmune thyroiditis (Hashimoto's)	Grossly lymphocytic and fibrotic thyrotoxicosis or hypothyroidism
Postpartum thyroiditis	Chronic lymphocytic thyroiditis, transient thyrotoxicosis or hypothyroidism
Riedel thyroiditis	Extensive fibrosis of the thyroid (p. 66)
Radiation thyroiditis	Radiation injury, transient thyrotoxicosis
Drug induced	Particularly with amiodarone

Table 6.2 Clinical presentation of thyroiditis

Form of thyroiditis	Clinical presentation	Thyroid function
Suppurative (acute)	Painful, tender thyroid, fever	Usually normal
Subacute (de Quervain)	Painful anterior neck, arthralgia, antecedent upper respiratory tract infection; generalized malaise.	Early thyrotoxicosis, occasionally late hypothyroidism
Autoimmune	Hashimoto's : goitre Atrophic: no goitre	Usually hypothyroid Sometimes euthyroid Rarely early thyrotoxicosis
Riedel	Hard woody consistency of thyroid	Usually normal

Chronic autoimmune (atrophic or Hashimoto's) thyroiditis

- *Subclinical autoimmune thyroiditis* Denotes the early stage of chronic thyroiditis. The thyroid gland is soft or firm and is usually normal in size or slightly enlarged. Thyroid function tests are normal.

- *Hashimoto's thyroiditis* Characterized by a painless, variably sized goitre with rubbery consistency and an irregular surface. The normal follicular structure of the gland is extensively replaced by lymphocytic and plasma cell infiltrates with formation of lymphoid germinal centres. The patient may have normal thyroid function or subclinical or overt hypothyroidism. Occasional patients present with thyrotoxicosis in association with a thyroid gland that is unusually firm and with high titres of circulating antithyroid antibodies.

- *Atrophic thyroiditis* Probably indicates endstage thyroid disease. These patients do not have goitre and are antibody positive. Biochemically, the picture is that of frank hypothyroidism.

Investigations

Investigations which are useful in establishing a diagnosis of Hashimoto's thyroiditis include:

- testing of thyroid function,

- thyroid antibodies (antithyroglobulin antibodies and antithyroperoxidase antibodies)

- occasionally a thyroid biopsy to exclude malignancy in patients who present with a goitre and dominant nodule.

Prognosis

The long-term prognosis of patients with chronic thyroiditis is good because hypothyroidism can easily be corrected with T_4 and the goitre is not usually of sufficient size to cause local symptoms. In the atypical situation where Hashimoto's thyroiditis presents with rapidly enlarging goitre and pain a short dose of prednisolone at a dose of 40 mg daily may prove helpful.

Any unusual increase in size of the thyroid in patients known to suffer from Hashimoto's thyroiditis should be investigated with FNAC since there is an association between this condition and thyroid lymphoma.

Other types of thyroiditis

Silent thyroiditis

Associated with transient thyrotoxicosis or hypothyroidism. A significant percentage of patients have personal or family history of autoimmune thyroid disease. It may progress to permanent hypothyroidism.

Postpartum thyroiditis (p. 506)

Thyroid dysfunction occurring within the first 6 months postpartum. Prevalence ranges from 5% to 7%. Postpartum thyroiditis develops in 30–52% of women who have positive thyroid peroxidase (TPO) antibodies. Most patients have a complete remission but some may progress to permanent hypothyroidism. It is twice as common in patients with Type I diabetes mellitus.

Chronic fibrosing (Riedel's) thyroiditis

A rare disorder characterized by intense fibrosis of the thyroid gland and surrounding structures leading to induration of the tissues of the neck. May be associated with mediastinal and retroperitoneal fibrosis, salivary gland fibrosis, sclerosing cholangitis, lachrymal gland fibrosis, and parathyroid gland fibrosis leading to hypoparathyroidism. Patients are usually euthyroid. Main differential diagnosis is thyroid neoplasia.

Management

Corticosteroids are usually ineffective. Tamoxifen is now the first line of treatment. Surgery may be required to relieve obstruction and to exclude malignancy.

Pyogenic thyroiditis

* Rare. Usually anteceded by a pyogenic infection elsewhere. Characterized by tenderness and swelling of the thyroid gland, redness and warmth of the overlying skin, and constitutional signs of infection.
* Piriform sinus should be excluded. Excision of tract is preferable to incision and drainage
* Treatment consists of antibiotic therapy and incision and drainage if a fluctuant area within the thyroid should occur.

Sub-acute thyroiditis (granulomatous, giant cell or de Quervain's thyroiditis)

+ Viral in origin.Symptoms include pronounced asthenia, malaise, pain over the thyroid or pain referred to lower jaw, ear, or occiput. Less commonly the onset is acute with fever, pain over the thyroid, and symptoms of thyrotoxicosis. Characteristically signs include exquisite tenderness and nodularity of the thyroid gland. There is characteristically an elevated ESR and a depressed radionuclide (^{99m}Tc can be used) uptake. Biochemically, the patient may be initially thyrotoxic though later the patient may become hypothyroid.

+ In mild cases, non-steroidal anti-inflammatory agents offer symptom relief. In severe cases glucocorticoids (prednisolone 20–40 mg/day) are effective. Propranolol can be used to control associated thyrotoxicosis. Treatment can be withdrawn when T_4 returns to normal. T_4 replacement is required if the patient becomes hypothyroid. Treatment with carbimazole or propylthiouracil is not indicated.

Further reading

Lazarus JH, Hall R, Othman S, Parkes AB, Richards CJ, McCulloch B, Harris B. The clinical spectrum of postpartum thyroid disease. *QJM* 1996; 89: 429–435.

Muller AF, Drexhage HA, Berghout A. Postpartum thyroiditis and autoimmune thyroiditis in women of child bearing age: recent insights and consequences for antenatal and postnatal care. *Endocrine Reviews* 2001; 22: 605–30.

Weetman AP. Autoimmune thyroid disease in *Endocrinology* ed DeGroot LJ and Jameson JL Vol. 2. WB Saunders & Co, Philadelphia, 2000.

Chapter 7
Hypothyroidism

Background

Hypothyroidism results from a variety of abnormalities that cause insufficient secretion of thyroid hormones. The commonest cause is autoimmune thyroid disease. *Myxoedema* is severe hypothyroidism in which there is accumulation of hydrophilic mucopolysaccharides in the ground substance of the dermis and other tissues leading to thickening of the facial features and doughy induration of the skin.

Table 7.1 Classification of the causes of hypothyroidism

	TSH	Free T$_4$
Non-goitrous	↑	↓
Postablative (radioiodine, surgery)		
Congenital development defect		
Atrophic thyroiditis		
Postradiation (e.g. for lymphoma)		
Goitrous	↑	↓
Chronic thyroiditis (Hashimoto's thyroiditis)		
Iodine deficiency		
Drug elicited (amiodarone, aminosalicylic acid, iodides, phenylbutazone, lithium)		
Heritable biosynthetic defects		
Maternally transmitted (antithyroid agents, iodides)		
Pituitary	↓	↓
Panhypopituitarism		
Isolated TSH deficiency		
Hypothalamic	↓	↓
Neoplasm		
Infiltrative (sarcoidosis)		
Congenital defects		
Infection (encephalitis)		
Self-limiting		
Following withdrawal of suppressive thyroid therapy		
Subacute thyroiditis and chronic thyroiditis with transient hypothyroidism		
Postpartum thyroiditis		

Clinical picture

Adult

- insidious non-specific onset
- fatigue, lethargy, constipation, cold intolerance, muscle stiffness, cramps, carpal tunnel syndrome, menorrhagia, later oligo- or amenorrhoea
- slowing of intellectual and motor activities
- decreasing appetite and weight gain
- dry skin; hair loss
- deep hoarse voice, decreasing visual acuity
- obstructive sleep apnoea

Myxoedema

- dull expressionless face, sparse hair, periorbital puffiness, macroglossia
- pale, cool skin that feels rough and doughy
- enlarged heart (dilation and pericardial effusion)
- megacolon/ intestinal obstruction
- cerebellar ataxia; psychiatric symptoms e.g. depression, psychosis
- prolonged relaxation phase of deep tendon reflexes
- peripheral neuropathy
- encephalopathy

Myxedema coma

- predisposed to by cold exposure, trauma, infection, administration of central nervous system depressants
- marked respiratory depression with increasing arterial P_{CO2}
- hyponatraemia from impaired water excretion and disordered regulation of vasopressin secretion/

Subclinical hypothyroidism

• This term is used to denote raised TSH levels in the presence of normal concentrations of free thyroid hormones. Treatment is indicated in patients with a past history of radioiodine treatment for thyrotoxicosis or positive thyroid antibodies as in these situations progression to overt hypothyroidism is almost inevitable (at least 5% per year of those with positive antithyroid peroxidase antibodies).

• There is controversy over the advantages of T_4 treatment in patients with negative thyroid antibodies and no previous radioiodine treatment.

• Some symptom scores have been shown to improve with T_4 treatment.

• There are concerns regarding the possible adverse effects in the form of reduced bone mineral density and increased risk of atrial fibrillation.

• Follow up with annual thyroid function tests is important.

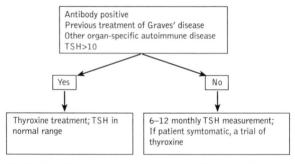

Fig. 7.1 Algorithm for management of subclinical hypothyroidism
Modified from Lindsay and Toft 1997; 349: 413–7.

Treatment of hypothyroidism

- Normal metabolic state should be restored gradually as rapid increase in metabolic rate may precipitate cardiac arrhythmias
- In the younger patients, start thyroxine at 100 μg. In the elderly, with a history of ischaemic heart disease, an initial dose of thyroxine 25–50 μg can be increased by 25 μg increments at 4 week intervals until normal metabolic state is attained.
- Optimum dose determined by clinical criteria and TSH measurements
- TSH should be checked only 2 months after any dose change. Once stabilized TSH should be checked on an annual basis.
- In patients with secondary hypothyroidism, free T_4 is the most useful parameter to follow.

Management of myxoedema coma

- Identify and treat concurrent precipitating illness.
- Antibiotic therapy after blood cultures.
- Management of hypothermia by passive external rewarming.
- Manage in intensive treatment unit if comatose. If not, nurse in a warm side room.
- Give warm humidified oxygen by facemask. Mechanical ventilation needed if hypoventilating.
- Aim for slow rise in core temperature (0.5° C/h).
- Cardiac monitor for supraventricular arrhythmias.
- Correct hyponatraemia (mild fluid restriction), hypotension (cautious volume expansion with crystalloid or whole blood), and hypoglycaemia (glucose administration).
- Monitor rectal temperature, oxygen saturation, BP, CVP, and urine output hourly.
- Take blood samples for thyroid hormones, TSH and cortisol before starting treatment. If hypocortisolaemic, administer glucocorticoids.
- Thyroid hormone replacement: no consensus has been reached. The following is an accepted regimen:
  - T_4 300–500 μg i/v or by nasogastric tube as a starting dose followed by 50–100 μg daily until oral medication can be taken
  - if no improvement within 24–48 h, T_3 10 μg i/v 8 hourly or 25 μg i/v 8 hourly can be given in addition to above.
- Give hydrocortisone 50–100 mg 6–8 hourly in case of cortisol deficiency.

Congenital hypothyroidism

Incidence: About 1 in 5000 neonates. All neonates should be screened.

Thyroid agenesis

Occurs 1 in 1800 births. In 80% cases the left lobe is affected. The remaining lobe is hypertrophied. There is no palpable tissue over the agenetic lobe

Thyroid hormone dysgenesis

* Caused by inborn errors of thyroid metabolism. The disorders are mostly autosomal recessive, indicating single protein defects.
* Can be caused by inactivation of the TSH receptor, abnormalities of the thyroid transcription factors TTF1, TTF2, and PAX8, or due to defects in iodide transport, organification (peroxidase), coupling, deiodinase, or thyroglobulin synthesis.
* In a large proportion of patients with congenital hypothyroidism, the molecular background is unknown.

Pendred's syndrome

Characterized by overt or subclinical hypothyroidism, goitre, and moderate to severe sensorineural hearing impairment. The prevalence varies between 1 in 15 000 and 1 in 100 000. There is a partial iodide organification defect detected by increased perchlorate discharge. Thyroid hormone synthesis is only mildly impaired and so may not be detected by neonatal thyroid screening.

Clinical features

The following features are late sequelae of congenital hypothyroidism and, with routine screening now available, should never be seen nowadays.

* physiological jaundice
* goitre
* hoarse cry, feeding problems, constipation, somnolence
* delay in reaching normal milestones of development; short stature
* coarse features with protruding tongue, broad flat nose, widely set eyes
* sparse hair and dry skin, protuberant abdomen with umbilical hernia
* impaired mental development, retarded bone age
* epiphyseal dysgenesis, delayed dentition.

Laboratory tests

- neonatal screening
- imaging procedure: ultrasonography or ^{123}I scintigraphy
- measurement of serum thyroglobulin and low molecular weight iodopeptides in urine to discriminate between the various types of defects.
- measurement of total urinary iodine excretion to differentiate inborn errors of metabolism from acquired transient forms of hypothyroidism due to iodine deficiency or iodine excess.

Treatment

Irrespective of the cause of congenital hypothyroidism, early treatment is essential to prevent cerebral damage. Sufficient T_4 should be given to maintain the TSH in the normal range.

Further reading

de Vijlder JJM, Vulsma T. In DeGroot LJ and Jameson JL (ed.) *Endocrinology,* Vol. 2, WB Saunders & Co, Philadelphia, 2000.

Chapter 8
Amiodarone and thyroid function

Background

- Amiodarone has a high concentration of iodine (39% by weight). It is a benzofuranic derivative and its structural formula closely resembles that of thyroxine. On a dose of Amiodarone between 200–600 mg daily, 7–21 mg iodine is made available each day. The optimal daily iodine intake is 150–200 µg. Amiodarone is distributed in several tissues from where it is slowly released. In one study terminal elimination half-life of amiodarone averaged 52.6 days with a standard deviation of 23.7 days.

- Abnormalities of thyroid function occur in up to 50% of patients (Table 8.2).

- In the UK and USA, 2% of patients on Amiodarone develop thyrotoxicosis and about 13% develop hypothyroidism.

- Patients residing in areas with high iodine intake develop amiodarone induced hypothyroidism (AIH) more often than amiodarone induced thyrotoxicosis (AIT), but AIT occurs more frequently in regions with low iodine intake.

- AIT can present several months after discontinuing the drug because of its long half-life.

- Hypothyroidism is commoner in women and in patients with thyroid autoantibodies.

- Thyroid function tests should be monitored every 6 months in patients taking amiodarone.

Pathogenesis

- The high iodine content of amiodarone may inhibit thyroid hormone synthesis and release causing AIH or leading to iodine-induced thyrotoxicosis.

- Thyrotoxicosis resulting from iodine excess and therefore increased hormone synthesis is referred to as *AIT type I*. Thyrotoxicosis due to a direct toxic effect of amiodarone is referred to as *AIT type II*. (Table 8.1).

- Drug-induced destructive thyroiditis results in leakage of thyroid hormones from damaged follicles into the circulation and like subacute thyroiditis can be followed by a transient hypothyroid state before euthyroidism is restored.

Table 8.1 Characteristics of AIT

	AIT type I	AIT type II
Aetiology	Iodine toxicity	Thyroiditis
Signs of clinical thyroid disease	Yes	No
Goitre	Frequent	Infrequent
Thyroid antibodies	Positive	Negative
Radioiodine uptake	Normal	Decreased
Thyroglobulin	Normal or slightly elevated	Very elevated
Serum IL6	Normal	Very elevated
Late hypothyroidism	No	Possible
Vascularity (Doppler)	Increased/normal	Reduced

Table 8.2 Thyroid function tests in clinically euthyroid patients after administration of amiodarone

Tests	1–3 months	>3 months
Free T_3	Decreased	Remains slightly decreased, but within normal range
TSH	Transient increase	Normal
Free T_4	Modest increase	Slightly increased compared to pre-treatment values, may be in normal range or slightly increased.
Reverse T_3	Increased	Increased

Table 8.3 Side effects and complications of amiodarone therapy

Side effect	Incidence (%)
Corneal microdeposits	100
Anorexia and nausea	80
Photosensitivity; Blue/grey skin discolouration	55–75
Ataxia, tremors, peripheral neuropathy	48
Deranged liver function tests	25
Abnormal thyroid function tests	14–18
Interstitial pneumonitis	10–13
Cardiac arrhythmias	2–3

Table 8.4 Treatment of amiodarone induced thyrotoxicosis

	Type 1 AIT	Type 2 AIT
Step 1 Aim: Restore euthyroidism	Carbimazole 30–40 mg/d or Propylthiouracil 300–400 mg/d in combination with potassium perchlorate 1 g/day for 16–40 days If possible discontinue amiodarone*	Discontinue amidarone if possible* Prednisolone 40 mg/day. In mixed forms add Carbimazole or propylthiouracil as in Type 1 AIT
Step 2: Definitive treatment	Radioiodine treatment or thyroidectomy	Follow up for possible spontaneous progression to hypothyroidism
*	If amiodarone cannot be withdrawn and medical therapy is unsuccessful, consider total thyroidectomy	If amiodarone cannot be withdrawn and medical therapy is unsuccessful, consider total thyroidectomy

Table 8.5 Treatment of amiodarone induced hypothyroidism

Underlying thyroid abnormality (Usually Hashimoto's thyroiditis)	Apparently normal thyroid
Amiodarone therapy can be continued. Add thyroxine replacement therapy.	• Discontinue amiodarone if possible and follow up for restoration of euthyroidism. Potassium perchlorate 1 g/day for 30 days to accelerate return to euthyroidism • If amiodarone cannot be withdrawn, start thyroxine replacement therapy

Treatment

+ Discontinuation of amiodarone does not always control the thyrotoxic state because of its long half-life (particularly in the obese).

+ The first line of treatment is ATDs (carbimazole or propylthiouracil).

+ Radioiodine is not usually effective because of reduced uptake by the thyroid gland.

+ Surgery remains a very successful form of treatment, with euthyroidism being restored within a matter of days. Achieving preoperative euthyroidism may be difficult, however.

+ Cardiac function may be compromised by propranolol used in combination with amiodarone, since this may produce bradycardia and sinus arrest.

+ A combination of corticosteroids and ATDs may be effective in AIT type II. A high dose of prednisolone, 40–60 mg daily, may be required for 8–12 weeks; studies where steroids have been discontinued after 2–3 weeks have been associated with a high relapse rate.

+ Potassium perchlorate inhibits iodide uptake by the thyroid gland, reduces intrathyroidal iodine, and renders thionomides more effective. It can be given as a 1 g daily dose together with carbimazole, a regime shown to restore euthyroidism in a large percentage of patients with both type I and type II AIT. In small case studies a combination of potassium perchlorate and carbimazole has been effective while treatment with amiodarone was continued.

+ After chronic administration a steady state is achieved. Thus in clinically euthyroid patients on amiodarone a slightly elevated T_4 is not indicative of hyperthyroidism, nor is a low T_3 indicative of hypothyroidism.

Further reading

Wiersinga WM (1997) Amiodarone and the thyroid. In Weetman AP, Grossman A (ed.) *Pharmacotherapeutics of Thyroid Gland*, Berlin: Springer-Verlag, pp. 225–287.

L Bartalena, S Brogioni, L Grasso, F Bogazzi, A Burelli, and E Martino. Treatment of amiodarone-induced thyrotoxicosis, a difficult challenge: results of a prospective study *J Clin Endocrinol Metab.* 1996; 81: 2930–2933.

Martino E, Bartalena L, Bogazzi F, Braverman LE. The Effects of Amiodarone on the Thyroid. *Endocrine Reviews* 2001; 22(2): 240–254.

Newman CM, Price A, Davies DW, Cray TA, Weetman AP. Amiodarone and the thyroid. *Heart* 1998; **79**: 121–127.

Chapter 9
Thyroid cancer

Epidemiology

- Clinically detectable thyroid cancer is rare. It accounts for <1% of all cancer and <0.5% of cancer deaths.
- Thyroid microcarcinoma (diameter <1 cm) may be found in multinodular goitres.
- Thyroid cancers are commonest in adults aged 40–50, and rare in children and adolescents.
- Women are affected more frequently than men.

Table 9.1 Classification of thyroid cancer

Cell of origin	Tumour type	Frequency (%)
Papillary	Differentiated	
	Papillary	70–80
	Follicular	15
	Undifferentiated (anaplastic)	6
C-cells	Medullary	5–10
Lymphocytes	Lymphoma	5–10

Table 9.2 Comparison of papillary, follicular and anaplastic carcinomas of the thyroid

Characteristic	Papillary Ca	Follicular Ca	Anaplastic Ca
Age at presentation	30–50 (mean 44)	40–50	60–80
Spread	Lymphatic	Haematogenous	Haematogenous
Prognosis	Good	Good	Poor
Treatment	Initially: near total thyroid-ectomy Postoperative TSH suppression High-risk patient: ^{131}I remnant ablation Postoperative total body radioiodine scan	Initially: near total thyroidectomy Postoperative TSH suppression ^{131}I remnant ablation Postoperative total body radioiodine scan	Total thyroidectomy with lymph node clearance Chemotherapy with adriamycin and cisplatin External beam irradiation

Aetiology

Irradiation

- There does not appear to be a threshold dose of external irradiation for thyroid carcinogenesis; doses of 200–500 cGy seem to produce thyroid cancer at a rate of about 0.5%/year.

- There is no evidence that therapeutic or diagnostic ^{131}I administration can induce thyroid cancer, although there is a small increase in death rates from thyroid cancer after ^{131}I. At present it is unclear whether this is due to an effect of ^{131}I or part of the natural history of the underlying thyroid disease.

- External irradiation at an age <20 years is associated with an increased risk of thyroid nodule development and thyroid cancer (most commonly papillary). The radioactive fallout from the Chernobyl nuclear explosion in 1986, resulted in a 4.7-fold increase in thyroid cancer in the regions of Belarus from 1985 to 1993, including a 34-fold increase in children. Most of these were papillary carcinomas.

- The risk is greater for women and when irradiation occurs at an younger age.

- There is a latency of at least 5 years with maximum risk at 20 years following exposure, though this was not seen following the Chernobyl disaster.

Other environmental factors

- Most investigators agree that iodine supplementation has resulted in a decrease in the incidence of follicular carcinoma.

Genetic syndromes and oncogenes

- *RET/PTC1* proto-oncogene abnormalities in the long arm of chromosome 10 are associated with some papillary tumours (5–30%), especially after irradiation (60–80%). It is similar to the abnormality associated with medullary thyroid carcinoma in MEN2A.

- 2 new protooncogenes have been have been identified: *RET/PTC2* and *RET/PTC3* TRK (less common).

- The tumour suppressor gene *p53* has been found to be mutated in dedifferentiated cancers.

- Overexpression of the *ras* oncogenes is found in papillary thyroid cancers and was found to be a marker for adverse prognosis in one study.

- c-*myc* mRNA expression has been correlated with histologic markers of papillary cancer aggression.
- PAX8-PPARγ1 may be useful in the diagnosis and treatment of thyroid carcinoma.

Papillary microcarcinoma of the thyroid (PMC)

- PMC is defined by WHO as a tumour focus of 1.0 cm or less in diameter. It is detected coincidentally on histopathological examination of the thyroid following resection of multinodular goitre.
- Autopsy studies show:
  - prevalence ranges from 1 to 35.6%
  - no significant difference in the prevalence rates of papillary microcarcinoma has been demonstrated between the sexes
  - PMC rarely progresses to clinically apparent thyroid cancer with advancing age
  - PMC can be multifocal
  - cervical lymphnode metastasis from PMC ranges from 4.3 to 18.2%
  - lymph node metastasis was most often associated with multifocal tumours.
- Although exposure to irradiation increases the likelihood of developing papillary thyroid cancer, the tumours will usually be >1.0 cm in diameter and thus not PMC.
- Follow-up studies suggest that PMC is a slow growing lesion which rarely spreads to distant sites and which carries a good prognosis.
- The recommendations for treatment of PMC vary widely:
  - The low morbidity and long survival mean that collection of randomized prospective data has never been performed and comparisons of therapies are based on retrospective studies.
  - The treatment of PMC should not cause more morbidity than the disease process itself.
  - Surgical treatment recommendations range from simple excision to ipsilateral lobectomy.
  - With adjuvant therapy the consensus is routine use of T_4 to suppress TSH, but not the use of radioiodine as there is no difference in the recurrence rate.

Papillary thyroid carcinoma

- constitutes almost 70% of all thyroid cancers
- commoner in women (3 : 1)
- rare in childhood, peaks occur in second and third decades and again in later life (bimodal frequency)
- incidence: 3–5 per 100 000 population.

Pathology

- Slow growing, usually non-encapsulated, may spread through the thyroid capsule to structures in the surrounding neck, especially regional lymph nodes. Multifocal in 30% of cases.
- Recognized variants are follicular, papillary, dorsal, columnar cell, tall cell, and diffuse sclerosing.
- *Histology* the tumour contains complex branching papillae that have a fibrovascular core covered by a single layer of tumour cells.
- Nuclear features include:
  - large size with pale staining, 'ground-glass' appearance (*orphan Annie-eye nucleus*).
  - deep nuclear grooves.
- The characteristic and pathognomic cytoplasmic feature is the 'psammoma body' which is a calcified, laminated, basophilic, stromal structure.
- It is confined to the neck in over 95% of cases, although 15–20% have local extra thyroidal invasion. Metastases (1–2% of patients) occur via lymphatics to local lymph nodes and more distantly to lungs.
- Several prognostic scoring systems are in use, none of which permits definitive decisions to be made for individual patients.

Management

Primary treatment: surgery

- Should be performed by an experienced thyroid surgeon at a centre with adequate case load to maintain surgical skills.
- In general, as near total thyroidectomy as possible should be performed.
- Clinically evident cervical lymph node metastasis is best treated with radical modified neck dissection with preservation of stern-

Adverse prognostic factors in papillary carcinoma (high-risk patients)

Thyroglobulin

+ A very sensitive marker of recurrence of thyroid cancer
+ Secreted by the thyroid tissue
+ After total thyroidectomy and radioactive iodine ablation, the levels of thyroglobulin should be <2 ng/L.
+ Measurement of thyroglobulin levels could be made difficult in the presence of antithyroglobulin antibodies.
+ There is controversy over whether the patient should come off T_4 or T_3 or be started on recombinant TSH before checking the thyroglobulin levels. Coming off thyroid hormones or giving TSH increases the sentivity of thyroglobulin to detect recurrence, but this may not effect survival rates.

Recurrent disease/distant metastases

+ In the case of recurrence, treatment employs all methods used in primary and adjuvant therapy.
+ Surgery for local metastases.
+ External radiotherapy is indicated in tumours that do not take up ^{131}I.
+ Bony and pulmonary metastases (usually osteolytic) may be treated with ^{131}I.
+ Unfortunately only 50% of metastases concentrate ^{131}I and bony metastases are often very difficult to irradiate.
+ Some advocate use of external beam radiation.
+ Response to chemotherapy is usually poor.

ocleidomastoid muscle, spinal accessory nerve, and internal jugular vein.

Adjuvant therapy: radioiodine therapy

* Postoperative radioiodine therapy is advised in the high-risk patient with differentiated thyroid cancer. After surgery in a low risk group, some thyroidologists argue that ^{131}I is not required. A dose of 3.1 GBq is used for thyroid ablation. A whole body scan done 4–6 months after administration of 150 MBq ^{131}I helps determine the presence of any residual disease. In the presence of metastasis a dose of approximately 5.5–7.4 GBq radioiodine is used. Liothyronine should be administered for 4–6 weeks in place of thyroxine. It is then omitted for 10 days prior to the scan, allowing TSH to rise. A low-iodine diet for 2 weeks increases the effective specific activity of the administered iodine.

* The patient should be isolated until residual dose meter readings indicate <30 MBq.

* Chronic suppression of serum TSH levels to <0.10 mU/l is standard practice in patients with differentiated thyroid carcinoma. Inhibition of TSH secretion reduces recurrence rate as TSH stimulates growth of the majority of thyroid cancer cells.

* Patients are followed up with thyroglobulin levels. After effective treatment thyroglobulin levels are undetectable. A trend of increasing thyroglobulin values should be investigated with a radioiodine uptake scan. Liothyronine (T_3) is substituted for T_4 4–6 weeks before the scan, and omitted for 10 days immediately beforehand.

Recombinant TSH

* Avoids morbidity of hypothyroidism during T_4 withdrawal.
* Useful for patients with TSH deficiency (hypopituitarism).
* Comparable thyroglobulin rise but reduced ^{131}I scan sensitivity compared to T_4 withdrawal.

Follicular carcinoma (FTC)

- constitutes 15% of all thyroid cancers
- mean patient age in most studies is 50 years
- commoner in women (2 : 1).
- relatively more common in endemic goitre areas.

Pathology

- Follicular carcinoma is a neoplasm of the thyroid epithelium that exhibits follicular differentiation and shows capsular or vascular invasion.
- Differentiation of benign follicular adenoma from encapsulated low-grade or minimally invasive tumours can be impossible to diagnose, particularly for the cytopathologist, and surgery is usually necessary for a follicular adenoma.
- FTC may be minimally invasive or widely invasive.
- Metastases (15–20% cases) are more likely to be spread by haematogenesis to the lung and bones and less likely to local lymph nodes.
- Hurthle cell carcinoma is an aggressive type of follicular tumour with a poor prognosis because it fails to concentrate ^{131}I.

Treatment

As for papillary thyroid carcinoma.

Follow-up of papillary and follicular thyroid carcinoma

- Follow-up usually involves an annual clinical review, with clinical examination for presence of suspicious lymph nodes and measurements of serum TSH (to ensure adequate TSH suppression to <0.1 mU/L) and thyroglobulin.

- Serum thyroglobulin should be undetectable in patients with total thyroid ablation. However, detectable levels may be seen for up to 6 months after thyroid ablation. A trend of increasing thyroglobulin level requires investigations with ^{131}I uptake scan (of thyroid hormones or with TSH stimulation) or any specific imaging modalities, such as CT scan of the lungs, or bone scans. Thyroglobulin antibodies must be checked, as there may be interactions with the thyroglobulin assays.

- Radioiodine scans are done annually for the first 3 years and if negative, not repeated unless there are clinical indications, like an increasing thyroglobulin level.

- Isolated lymph node metastases can occasionally be associated with normal thyroglobulin. Stopping thyroid hormone replacement before the measurement of thyroglobulin can increase sensitivity of detecting persistent recurrent disease.

- Detectable thyroglobulin and absent uptake on radioiodine uptake scan may be due to dedifferentiation of the tumour and failure to take up iodine. A PET scan may be useful in this situation. If a PET scan is not available, an iodine uptake scan following 150 MBq ^{131}I can be useful.

Thyroid cancer in children

- Uncommon, with an incidence of 0.2–5 per million per year.
- >85% are papillary, but with more aggressive behaviour than in adults (local invasion and distant metastases are commoner).
- Recently an increased incidence in children in Belarus and Ukraine has been reported following the Chernobyl nuclear accident in 1986. RET oncogene rearrangements are common in these tumours.
- Management is similar to adults, with a similar controversy as to the extent of initial surgery.
- Various studies report an overall recurrence rate of 0–39%; disease-free survival of 80–93%, and disease-specific mortality of 0–10%.
- Evidence is currently lacking on the independent risks or benefits of radioactive iodine or extensive surgery.
- Many investigators recommend lifelong follow-up with a combination of thyroglobulin and radionuclide scanning.

Thyroid cancer and pregnancy

- The natural course of thyroid cancer developing during pregnancy may be different from that in non-pregnant women.
- Any woman presenting with a thyroid nodule in pregnancy appears to have an increased risk for thyroid cancer.
- Evaluation should be undertaken with FNAC. Radioiodine scan is contraindicated.
- Lesions <2 cm diameter or any lesion appearing after 24 weeks gestation should be treated with TSH suppression and further evaluations carried out postpartum.
- If FNAC is suspicious or diagnostic, operation should be performed at the earliest safe opportunity – generally the second trimester or immediately postpartum.
- ^{131}I ablation should be scheduled for the postpartum period and the mother advised to stop breast-feeding.
- Avoid pregnancy for 6 months after any ^{131}I ablation.

Medullary thyroid carcinoma (MTC)

See section on MEN (Chapters 96 and page 717).

Anaplastic (undifferentiated) thyroid cancer

- Rare.
- Peak incidence: 7th decade. F : M = 1 : 1.5.
- Characterized by rapid growth of a firm/hard fixed tumour.
- Often infiltrates local tissue such as larynx and great vessels and so does not move on swallowing. Stridor and obstructive respiratory symptoms are common.
- Aggressive, with poor long term prognosis – 7% 5 year survival rate and a mean survival of 6 months from diagnosis.
- Optimal results occur following total thyroidectomy. This is usually not possible and external irradiation is used, sometimes in association with chemotherapy.

Lymphoma

- Uncommon
- Almost always associated with autoimmune thyroid disease (Hashimoto's thyroiditis). Occurs more commonly in women and in patients aged >40 years.
- Characterized by rapid enlargement of the thyroid gland.
- May be limited to thyroid gland or part of a more extensive systemic lymphoma (usually non-Hodgkin's lymphoma). Trucut biopsy may be required.
- Treatment with radiotherapy alone or chemotherapy if more extensive often produces good results.

Further reading

Ain KB. Papillary thyroid carcinoma: Aetiology, Assessment and therapy; *Endocrinology and Metabolism Clinics of North America* 1995; 24(4): 711–760.

Grebe SK, Hay ID. Follicular thyroid cancer. *Endocrinology and Metabolism Clinics of North America* 1995; 24(4): 761–802.

Kroll TG, Sarraf P, Pecciarini L, Chen CJ, Mueller E, Spiegelman BM, Fletcher JA. PAX8-PPAR gamma1 fusion oncogene in human thyroid carcinoma *Science* 2000; 289(5483): 1357–1360.

Mazzaferri EL, Jhiang SM. Long term impact of initial surgery and medical therapy on follicular and papillary cancer. *American Journal of Medicine* 1998

Wartofsky L, Sherman SI, Gopal J, Schlumberger M, Hay ID. The use of radioactive iodine in patients with papillary and follicular thyroid cancer. *Journal of Clinical Endocrinology Metabolism* 1998; 83: 4195–420.

Part II
Pituitary

Chapter 10
Anatomy and physiology of anterior pituitary gland

Anatomy

The pituitary gland is situated in the pituitary fossa. Below is the sphenoid air sinus, on either side the internal carotid artery and cavernous sinus, and above the posterior pituitary is continuous with the pituitary stalk of the basal hypothalamus, which with the pituitary portal vessels passes down through the dura mater which roofs the pituitary fossa.

The posterior pituitary gland is supplied by the inferior hypophyseal branches of the internal carotid artery, and the anterior pituitary gland by the hypothalamohypophyseal portal veins.

Physiology

Prolactin (PRL) secretion*

Pulsatile secretion in a circadian rhythm with around 14 pulses/24 h, and a superimposed bimodal 24 h pattern of secretion, with a nocturnal peak during sleep and a lesser peak in the evening.

Growth hormone (GH) secretion*

Pulsatile – GH is usually undetectable in the serum apart from 5–6 90 min pulses/24 h that occur more commonly at night.

LH/FSH secretion

Glycoprotein hormone, with a chain common to LH, FSH (also TSH and hCG), but ß chain specific for each hormone. Pulsatile secretion.

Thyroid stimulating hormone (TSH) secretion

Pulsatile, with 9 ± 3 pulses/24 h, and increased amplitude of pulses at night.

Adrenocorticotrophic hormone (ACTH)*

- Single-chain polypeptide cleaved from pro-opiomelanocortin (POMC).
- Circadian rhythm of secretion, beginning to rise from 3 a.m. to a peak before waking in the morning, and falling thereafter.

---

*Concentrations increased with stress: NB venepuncture.

Chapter 11
Imaging

Background

- Magnetic resonance imaging (MRI) currently provides the optimal imaging of the pituitary gland.
- Computed tomography (CT) scans may still be useful in demonstrating calcification in tumours (e.g. craniopharyngiomas) and hyperostosis in association with meningiomas, or evidence of bone destruction.
- Plain skull radiography may show evidence of pituitary fossa enlargement but has been superseded by MRI.

MRI appearances

- T1 weighted images demonstrate cerebrospinal fluid (CSF) as dark grey, and brain as much whiter. This imaging is useful for demonstrating anatomy clearly. The normal posterior pituitary gland appears bright white (due to neurosecretory granules and phospholipids) on T1 weighted images, in contrast to the anterior gland which is of the same signal as white matter. The bony landmarks have low signal intensity on MRI, and air in the sphenoid sinus below the fossa shows no signal. Fat in the dorsum sellae may shine white. T2 weighted images may sometimes be used to characterize haemisoderin and fluid contents of a cyst.
- Intravenous gadolinium compounds are used for contrast enhancement. Because the pituitary and pituitary stalk have no blood–brain barrier, in contrast to the rest of the brain, the normal pituitary gland enhances brightly following gadolinium injection. Particular uses are the demonstration of cavernous sinus involvement and microadenomas.
- The normal pituitary gland has a flat or slightly concave upper surface. In adolescence or pregnancy, the surface may become slightly convex.

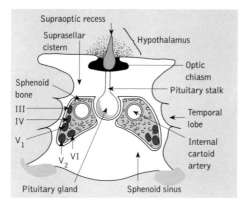

Reproduced from *Oxford Textbook of Medicine*, 3rd edn. With permission.

Pituitary adenomas

On T1 weighted images, pituitary adenomas are of lower signal intensity than the remainder of the normal gland. The size and extent of the pituitary adenomas are noted in addition to the involvement of other structures such as invasion of the cavernous sinus, erosion of the fossa, and relations to the optic chiasm. Larger tumours may show low intensity areas compatible with necrosis or cystic change, or higher intensity signal due to haemorrhage. The presence of microadenomas may be difficult to demonstrate. Contrast enhancement may assist, as may asymmetry of the gland or stalk position.

Craniopharyngiomas

These appear as suprasellar (occasionally intrasellar) masses with cystic and/or calcified portions.

Further reading

Naidich MJ, Russell EJ. Current approaches to imaging of the sellar region and pituitary. *Endocrinology and Metabolism Clinics of N America* 1999; 28: 45.

Chapter 12
Pituitary function: dynamic tests

Insulin tolerance test (ITT)

Indications
* assessment of ACTH reserve
* assessment of GH reserve.

Physiology
Intravenous insulin is used to induce hypoglycaemia (glucose <2.2 mmol/L with signs of glycopenia) which produces a standard stress causing ACTH and GH secretion.

Contraindications
* basal cortisol <100 nmol/L
* untreated hypothyroidism
* abnormal ECG
* ischaemic heart disease
* seizures
* NB Patients should discontinue oestrogen replacement for 6 weeks before the test as increased CBG will make the cortisol results difficult to interpret.

Procedure
* Continued medical surveillance is essential throughout.
* Patient is fasted overnight. Weight is checked.
* Insert cannula. Check basal (time 0) glucose, cortisol, and GH.
* Administer intravenous soluble insulin 0.15 U/kg (occasionally 0.3 U/kg needed in untreated Cushing's syndrome and acromegaly because of increased insulin resistance).
* Measure glucose, GH, and cortisol at 30, 45, 60, 90 and 120 min. Repeat insulin dose if a stick test for glucose does not show hypoglycaemia at 45 min.
* Test is terminated if prolonged hypoglycaemia – may need to administer 25 mL of 25% dextrose and i/v 100 mg hydrocortisone after sampling for cortisol and GH.
* Ensure patient eats lunch and has normal glucose before discharge.

Response
* The normal response is for glucose to fall to <2.2 mmol/L, and for cortisol to rise to >580 nmol/L and GH to >20 mU/L.

- In the presence of inadequate hypoglycaemia, the test cannot be interpreted.

- A normal cortisol response demonstrates ability to withstand stress (including major surgery) without requiring glucocorticoid cover.

- A subnormal response in an asymptomatic patient (e.g. peak cortisol 450–580 nmol/L) may be managed by administration of glucocorticoids at time of stress only.

- Other patients with subnormal responses require glucocorticoid replacement treatment (see p. 121).

- A GH response less than 10 mU/L is indicative of severe GH deficiency and in the appropriate clinical situation (see p. 124) GH replacement therapy may be recommended. Values between 10 and 20 are borderline.

Glucagon test

Indications

* assessment of ACTH reserve
* assessment of GH reserve.

Physiology

Glucagon leads to release of insulin which then leads to GH and ACTH release. The response may be secondary to the drop in glucose seen after the initial rise following glucagon injection, or may relate to the nausea induced by glucagon.

Contraindications

* Often unreliable in patients with diabetes mellitus.
* NB Patients should discontinue oestrogen replacement for 6 weeks before the test as increased CBG will make the cortisol results difficult to interpret.

Procedure

The test is performed at 9 a.m. following an overnight fast. Basal GH and cortisol are measured then 1 mg (1.5 mg if patient weighs >90 kg) glucagon is administered s/c. Samples for GH, cortisol, and glucose are checked from 90 min every 30 min till 240 min.

Response

* The normal response is a rise in glucose to a maximum at 90 min. Cortisol rises to >580 nmol/L and GH rises to >20 mU/L.
* This is a less reliable test than the ITT as 20% normal individuals may fail to respond.

ACTH stimulation test

Short synacthen test.

Indication

* assessment of adrenal cortical function
* assessment of ACTH reserve

Physiology

Low cortisol that does not rise following administration of ACTH demonstrates adrenal cortical disease. Prolonged ACTH administration will lead to cortisol secretion in ACTH deficiency but not in primary adrenal disease. It *can* be used to assess ACTH reserve, as in ACTH deficiency the adrenal cortex is unable to respond to a stimulatory signal within 30 minutes. (See p. 117)

Procedure

* The test can be done at any time of the day; the response is not time dependent.
* Synacthen is administered 250 μg i/m, and cortisol measured at 0, 30, and 60 min. When this test is used to measure ACTH reserve, only the 0 and 30 min values are required. The dose may also be given i/v with identical results.
* NB Patients should discontinue oestrogen replacement for 6 weeks before the test as increased CBG will make the cortisol results difficult to interpret.

Response

The post-stimulation cortisol should rise to >580 nmol/L at 30 min. This is an unreliable test of ACTH reserve within 6 weeks of an insult e.g. surgery to the pituitary.

Note Since 250 mcg synacthen is a supra-physiological stimulus, some investigators recommend the use of 1 mcg (low dose short synacthen)

Arginine test

Indication
Second line test for assessment of GH reserve.

Physiology
Arginine leads to GH release.

Contraindications
None

Procedure
- Fast from midnight, and administer 0.5 g/kg (max 30 g) arginine i/v in 100 mL normal saline over 30 min from time 0 (9 a.m.).
- Sample glucose and GH at 0, 30, 60, 90, and 120 min.

Response
A normal response is a rise in GH to >15–20 mU/L.

Clomiphene test

Indications

Assessment of gonadotrophin deficiency (e.g. Kallmann's syndrome).

Physiology

Clomiphene has mixed oestrogen and antioestrogenic effects. The basis of the test is competitive inhibition of oestrogen binding at the hypothalamus and pituitary gland, leading to increased LH and FSH after 3 days.

Contraindications

* Avoid in those with liver disease.
* May transiently worsen depression.

Procedure

* Advise patient of possible side-effects – visual disturbance (peripheral flickering of vision), and also of possible ovulation in women (contraceptive advice).
* Measure LH and FSH on days 0, 4, 7, and 10. In women measure day 21 progesterone to detect whether ovulation has occurred.
* Administer clomiphene 3 mg/kg (max 200 mg/day) in divided doses for 7 days.

Response

* The normal response is a doubling of gonadotrophins by day 10, usually rising beyond the normal range.
* In hypothalamic disease no gonadotropin rise is seen. Pre-pubertal patients may show a fall in gonadotrophins.
* Ovulation is presumed if day 21 progesterone is >30 nmol/L.

hCG test

Indications

To examine Leydig cell function, see p. 437.

GnRH test

Indication
Assessment of LH/FSH reserve

Physiology
Synthetic GnRH leads to pituitary gland release of FSH and LH.

Contraindications
None

Procedure
- Because of variations through the menstrual cycle, this is usually performed in women during the follicular phase if patients are cycling.
- Sample LH and FSH 0, 20, and 60 min after administration of GnRH.

Response
- LH levels rise quickly to peak at 20 min whereas FSH levels are maximal at 60 min.
- This test does not diagnose gonadotrophin deficiency, as subnormal, normal, or exaggerated responses may be seen. It demonstrates the amount of pituitary reserve of LH/FSH secretion. It is now rarely used.
- Occasional patients with acromegaly have a GH response

TRH test

This is rarely required with currently available sensitive TSH assays.

Indications

- Differentiation of pituitary TSH and hypothalamic TRH deficiency.
- Differentiation of TSH-secreting tumour from thyroid hormone resistance (Table 3.5, p. 48).
- Diagnosis of hyperthyroidism (largely superseded by sensitive TSH assay).

Procedure

- Administer TRH 200 µg i/v to supine patient.
- Measure T_4 and TSH at time 0, and TSH at 20 and 60 min.
- Note occasional reports of pituitary tumour haemorrhage. TRH induces a rise in blood pressure.

Response

- Normal response is rise in TSH by more than 2 mU/L to >3.4 mU/L, with a maximum at 20 min and lower values at 60 min.
- A delayed peak (60 min rather than 20 min) is typically found in hypothalamic disease.
- In hyperthyroidism there is no TSH response to TRH.
- The TRH test is also used rarely in investigation of hyper-prolactinaemia and acromegaly (see pp. 140 and 149)

Chapter 13
Hypopituitarism

Definition

Hypopituitarism refers to either partial or complete deficiency of anterior and/or posterior pituitary hormones, and may be due to primary pituitary disease or to hypothalamic pathology which interferes with the hypothalamic control of the pituitary.

Causes

* pituitary tumours
* parapituitary tumours (craniopharyngiomas, meningiomas, secondary deposits (breast, lung), chordomas, gliomas)
* radiotherapy (pituitary, cranial, nasopharyngeal)
* pituitary infarction (apoplexy), Sheehan's syndrome
* infiltration of the pituitary gland (sarcoidosis, lymphocytic hypophysitis, haemochromatosis, Langerhans cell histiocytosis)
* empty sella
* infection (tuberculosis, pituitary abscess)
* trauma
* isolated hypothalamic releasing hormone deficiency (e.g. Kallmann's syndrome due to GnRH deficiency).

Apoplexy

Apoplexy refers to infarction of the pituitary gland due to either haemorrhage or ischaemia. It occurs most commonly in patients with pituitary adenomas, usually macroadenomas, but other pre-disposing conditions include postpartum (Sheehan's syndrome), radiation therapy, diabetes mellitus, anticoagulant treatment, reduction in intracranial pressure.

It may present with a syndrome which is difficult to differentiate from any other intracranial haemorrhage with sudden onset headache, vomiting, meningism, and visual disturbance and cranial nerve palsy. The diagnosis is based on the clinical features and pituitary imaging which shows high signal on T1 and T2 weighted images (see the section on imaging). It has been suggested that early surgery (within 8 days) provides the optimal chance for neurological recovery. However, some patients may be managed conservatively if the patient has no significant visual or other neurological loss.

Empty sella syndrome

An enlarged pituitary fossa, which may be primary (due to arach-noid herniation through a congenital diaphragmatic defect) or secondary to surgery, radiotherapy, or pituitary infarction. The majority of patients have normal pituitary function. Hypo-pituitarism (and or hyperprolactinaemia) is found in <10%. A radiologically empty sella may rarely be associated with a func-tioning pituitary tumour.

Sheehan's syndrome

Haemorrhagic infarction of the enlarged postpartum pituitary gland following severe hypotension usually due to blood loss, e.g. postpartum haemorrhage. Improvement in obstetric care has made this a rare occurrence in the developed world.

Features

- The clinical features depend on the severity of pituitary hormone deficiency and the rate of development, in addition to whether there is intercurrent illness. In the majority of cases, the development of hypopituitarism follows a characteristic order, with secretion of GH, then gonadotrophins being affected first followed by TSH and ACTH secretion at a later stage. PRL deficiency is rare, except in Sheehan's syndrome associated with failure of lactation. ADH deficiency is virtually unheard of with pituitary adenomas, but may be seen rarely with infiltrative disorders and trauma.

- The majority of the clinical features are similar to those occurring when there is target gland insufficiency. There are important differences – e.g. lack of pigmentation and normokalaemia in ACTH deficiency in contrast to increased pigmentation and hyperkalaemia (due to aldosterone deficiency) in Addison's disease.

- NB *Houssay phenomenon* amelioration of diabetes mellitus in patients with hypopituitarism due to reduction in counter-regulatory hormones.

Table 13.1 Summary of clinical features of hypopituitarism

Hormone deficiency	Clinical features
GH	Adult GHD (see p. 123)
	Reduced exercise capacity, reduced lean body mass, impaired psychological well-being, increased cardiovascular risk
LH/FSH	Anovulatory cycles, oligo/amenorrhoea, dyspareunia in women
	Erectile dysfunction and testicular atrophy in males
	Reduced libido, infertility and loss of secondary sexual hair (often after many years) in both sexes
ACTH	As in Addison's disease, except lack of hyperpigmentation, absence of hyperkalaemia (p. 312)
TSH	As in primary hypothyroidism (see p. 71)
PRL	Failure of lactation
ADH	Polyuria and polydipsia

Investigation

The aims of investigation of hypopituitarism are to biochemically assess the extent of pituitary hormone deficiency and also to elucidate the cause.

Basal hormone levels

Basal concentrations of the anterior pituitary hormone as well as the target organ hormone should be measured, as the pituitary hormones may remain within the normal range despite low levels of target hormone. Measurement of the pituitary hormone alone does not demonstrate that the level is inappropriately low, and the diagnosis may be missed.

- LH and FSH, and testosterone (9 a.m.) or oestradiol
- TSH and thyroxine
- 9 a.m. cortisol
- PRL
- IGF-1 (NB May be normal in up to half of GHD depending on age).

Dynamic tests

- Dynamic tests, such as the insulin tolerance test (ITT) (p. 104) or glucagon test (p. 106) if the ITT is contraindicated, are used to assess cortisol and GH reserve.
- Some centres use the short synacthen test to assess ACTH reserve using the 0 and 30 min values of cortisol (p. 107). There are few false negatives using this investigation, and it is simpler to perform than the former tests but gives no measure of GH reserve. It is important to note that falsely normal results occur when hypopituitarism is of recent onset because the test relies on the fact that ACTH deficiency causes atrophy of the adrenal cortex and therefore a delayed response to synacthen. Less than 6 weeks of ACTH deficiency may allow a 'normal' adrenal response.

Posterior pituitary function

- It is important to assess and replace corticotroph function before assessing posterior pituitary hormone production because ACTH deficiency leads to reduced GFR and the inability to excrete a water load, which may therefore mask diabetes insipidus (DI).

• Plasma and urine osmolality are often adequate as baseline measures. However, in patients suspected to have DI, a formal water deprivation test should usually be performed (see p. 235).

Investigation of the cause

• Pituitary imaging – MRI ± contrast
• Investigation of hormonal hypersecretion if a pituitary tumour is demonstrated.
• Investigation of infiltrative disorders as discussed in Chapter 27, e.g. serum and CSF ACE, ferritin, hCG.
• Occasionally biopsy of the lesion is required.

Treatment

Treatment involves adequate and appropriate hormone replacement (see chapters 14, 15 and 33), and management of the underlying cause.

Isolated defects of pituitary hormone secretion

Rarely, patients have isolated insufficiency of only one anterior pituitary hormone. The aetiology of these disorders is largely unknown, although loss of hypothalamic control may play a role; an autoimmune pathology has been suggested in some and genetic mutations in others

• GnRH deficiency (Kallman's syndrome – congenital GnRH deficiency ± anosmia)
• isolated ACTH deficiency
• Pit-1 gene mutation (leads to isolated GH, PRL, and TSH deficiency)
• Prop-1 gene mutation (leads to isolated GH, PRL, TSH and gonadotrophin deficiency).

Chapter 14
Anterior pituitary hormone replacement

Background

Anterior pituitary hormone replacement therapy is usually performed by replacing the target hormone rather than the pituitary or hypothalamic hormone that is actually deficient. The exceptions to this are GH replacement (discussed on p. 123) and when fertility is desired (p. 474).

Table 14.1 Usual doses of hormone replacement therapy

Hydrocortisone	10 mg on waking, 5 mg at lunch time, and 5 mg early evening or twice daily regimens with a total dose of 15–30 mg/d
or	
Prednisolone	4 mg on waking and 2 mg early evening (total dose 5–7.5 mg/d)
Thyroxine	100–150 µg/d
GH	0.2–0.6 mg/d (0.4–1.5 IU)
Oestrogens/testosterone	Depends on formulation

Thyroid hormone replacement

This is discussed in the section on primary hypothyroidism (p. 79).

Monitoring of therapy

In contrast to replacement in primary hypothyroidism, the measurement of TSH cannot be used to assess adequacy of replacement in TSH deficiency due to hypothalamopituitary disease. Therefore, monitoring of treatment in order to avoid under- and over-replacement should be via both clinical assessment and by measuring Free thyroid hormone concentrations.

Sex hormone replacement

See pp. 405 and 439. Oestrogen/testosterone administration is the usual method of replacement, but gonadotrophin therapy is required if fertility is desired (see p. 480).

Glucocorticoids

Replacement therapy

Patients with ACTH deficiency usually need glucocorticoid replacement only and do not require mineralocorticoids, in contrast to patients with Addison's disease (p. 318).

The glucocorticoid most commonly used for replacement therapy is *hydrocortisone*. It is rapidly absorbed with a short half-life (90–120 min). *Prednisolone* and *dexamethasone* can occasionally be used for glucocorticoid replacement. The longer half-lives of these two drugs makes them useful where sustained ACTH suppression is required in, for example, congenital adrenal hyperplasia (CAH). Dexamethasone is useful when monitoring endogenous production as it is not detected in most cortisol assays. Cortisol acetate was previously used for glucocorticoid replacement therapy but requires hepatic conversion to the active cortisol.

Monitoring of replacement

This is important to avoid over-replacement which is associated with increased blood pressure, elevated glucose and insulin, and reduced bone mineral density (BMD). Under-replacement leads to the non-specific symptoms as seen in Addison's disease (p. 314). A clinical assessment is important but biochemical monitoring using plasma and urine cortisol (UFC) measurements are used by most endocrinologists. The aim is to keep the UFC within the reference range (<220 nmol/24 h). Many centres use plasma cortisol measurements on a hydrocortisone day curve. The aim is to keep the plasma cortisol between 150 and 300 nmol/L, avoiding nadirs of <50 nmol/L pre-doses.

Safety

Patients should be encouraged to wear a Medic-Alert indicating that they are cortisol deficient, to carry a steroid card, and to keep a vial of parenteral hydrocortisone at home to be administered in emergency situations.

Equivalent oral glucocorticoid doses

Prednisolone 5 mg is approximately equivalent to

* hydrocortisone 20 mg
* dexamethasone 0.75 mg
* methylprednisolone 4 mg.

Acute/severe intercurrent illness

* *Mild disease without fever* No change in glucocorticoid replacement.
* *Pyrexial illness* Double replacement dose (e.g. hydrocortisone 20, 10, 10 mg) for duration of fever.
* *Vomiting or diarrhoea* Parenteral therapy 100 mg i/m (from GP/trained relative; useful for patient to have vial of hydrocortisone at home with instruction sheet for emergency administration by suitable trained personnel).
* *Severe illness/operation* Parenteral therapy with i/m hydrocortisone 50–100 mg 6 hourly (e.g. 72 h for major surgery, 24 h for minor surgery).

Hydrocortisone day curve

There are various protocols for this test ranging from a three-point curve to detect under-replacement (used with 24 h UFC to detect over-replacement) – serum cortisol checked at 9. a.m., 12.30 p.m. (before the lunch time dose), and 5 p.m. (pre evening dose), to more frequent sampling to detect over and under-replacement. This involves serum cortisol at time 0, then administration of the morning dose of hydrocortisone. Plasma cortisol is then checked at 30 min, 1 h, 2, 3, and 5 h (prelunchtime dose specimen), and 7 and 9 h (pre evening dose) followed by samples at 10 and 11 h.

* Oral oestrogen therapy should be stopped 6 weeks before the test as increased CBG leading to higher cortisol values will make the test uninterpretable.
* This test is only valid for hydrocortisone replacement. Prednisolone or dexamethasone replacement can only be monitored clinically.

Chapter 15
Growth hormone replacement therapy in adults

Background

There is now a considerable amount of evidence that there are significant and specific consequences of GH deficiency (GHD) in adults, and that many of these features improve with GH replacement therapy. GH replacement for adults has now been approved in many countries.

Definition

It is important to differentiate between adult and childhood onset GHD.

- Although *childhood onset* GHD occurs secondary to structural lesions such as craniopharyngiomas and germinomas, and following treatment such as cranial irradiation, the commonest cause in childhood is an isolated variable deficiency of GH releasing hormone (GHRH) which may resolve in adult life because of maturation of the hypothalamo-somatotroph axis. It is therefore important to retest patients with childhood onset GHD when linear growth is completed (50% recovery of this group).

- *Adult onset* GHD usually occurs secondary to a structural pituitary or parapituitary condition or due to the effects of surgical treatment or radiotherapy.

Prevalence

- adult onset GHD 1/10 000
- adult GHD due to adult and childhood onset GHD 3/10 000.

Benefits of GH replacement

- Improved quality of life and psychological well-being.
- Improved exercise capacity.
- Increased lean body mass and reduced fat mass.
- Prolonged GH replacement therapy (more than 12–24 months) has been shown to increase BMD, which would be expected to reduce fracture rate.
- There are as yet no outcome studies in terms of cardiovascular mortality. However, GH replacement does lead to a reduction (approximately 15%) in cholesterol. GH replacement also leads to improved ventricular function and increased left ventricular mass.

Diagnosis

The diagnosis of GHD depends on appropriate biochemical testing in the presence of an appropriate clinical context. The latter is important, because distinguishing 'partial GHD' from physiological causes of reduced GH secretion such as obesity or ageing and pathological causes, e.g. hypercortisolaemia in Cushing's syndrome, can be problematic. In these situations GHD can be diagnosed when there is supportive evidence such as pituitary disease and other anterior pituitary hormone deficiencies.

Who should be tested?

As the features of GHD may be non-specific, and biochemical tests can be misleading in certain clinical situations such as obesity, investigation of GHD should only be performed in the following groups of patients:

- Patients with hypothalamo-pituitary disease (GHD occurs early in hypopituitarism, and is almost invariable in patients with other anterior pituitary hormone deficiencies).
- Patients who had childhood onset GHD.
- Patients who have received cranial irradiation.

Investigation of GH deficiency

Dynamic tests of GH secretion

- ITT most widely used test. Peak GH <10 mU/L (3 μg/L) are diagnostic of GHD. GH values of 10–20 mU/L indicate partial GHD.

- Alternative tests if the ITT is contraindicated include a combination of GHRH and GH releasing peptide-6 (GHRP-6), glucagon, arginine stimulation tests, or arginine in combination with GHRH. The clonidine test, although useful in paediatric practice, is not helpful in the diagnosis of adult GHD. The recently described natural ligand for the GHRH receptor GHrelin may prove useful in the future. Further validation of these newer tests and determination of cut-off values is required.

- A second confirmatory dynamic biochemical test is recommended, particularly in patients who have suspected isolated GH deficiency. A single GH dynamic test is sufficient to diagnose GHD in patients with two or three pituitary hormonal defects.

IGF-1

IGF-1 concentrations may remain within the age-matched reference range despite severe GHD in up to 50% of patients, and therefore does not exclude the diagnosis, and reduced IGF-1 is seen in a number of conditions.

Investigations in adult GH deficiency

* stimulated GH below 10 mU/L (3 μg/L)
* low or low–normal IGF-1 (IGF-1 may be normal in up to 50%, depending on age)
* decreased BMD
* increased insulin resistance
* hyperlipidaemia (increased LDL)
* impaired cardiac function.

Causes of lowered IGF-1 levels

* GHD
* malnutrition
* poorly controlled diabetes mellitus
* hepatic disease
* renal disease
* severe intercurrent illness.

Clinical features of GH deficiency

* impaired well-being
* reduced energy and vitality (depressed mood, increased social isolation, increased anxiety)
* reduced muscle mass and impaired exercise capacity
* increased central adiposity (increased waist : hip ratio) and increased total body fat
* decreased sweating and impaired thermogenesis
* increased cardiovascular risk
* increased fracture risk (osteoporosis).

Treatment of GH deficiency

All patients with GHD should be considered for GH replacement therapy. In particular, patients with impaired quality of life, reduced mineral density, an adverse cardiovascular risk profile, and reduced exercise capacity should be considered for treatment.

Dose

• Unlike paediatric practice, where GH doses are determined by body weight and surface area, most adult endocrinologists use dose titration using serial IGF-1 measurements to increase the dose of GH until the IGF-1 approaches the middle to upper end of the age-matched IGF-1 reference range. This reduces the likelihood of side-effects, mainly related to fluid retention, which were frequently observed in the early studies of GH replacement in adults when doses equivalent to those used in paediatric practice were used.

• The normal production of GH is 0.2–0.5 mg/day in an adult. Current recommendations are a starting dose of 0.1–0.4 mg/d. The maintenance dose is usually 0.2–0.6 mg/d. The dose in women is often higher than for age-matched men.

Monitoring of treatment

• A clinical examination, looking for reduction in overall body weight (a good response is loss of 3–5 kg in 12 months), and reduced waist to hip ratio. Blood pressure may fall in hypertensive patients because of reduction in peripheral systemic vascular resistance.

• IGF-1 is monitored to avoid over-replacement, aiming to keep values within the age-matched reference range. During dose titration, IGF-1 should be measured every 1–2 months. Once a stable dose is reached, IGF-1 should be checked at least once a year.

• The adverse effects experienced with GH replacement usually resolve with dose reduction, and tend to be less frequent with the lower starting doses used in current practice.

• GH treatment may be associated with impairment of insulin sensitivity, and therefore markers of glycaemia should be monitored.

• Lipids should be monitored annually. Bone mineral density should be monitored every 2 years, particularly in those with reduced BMD.

• It may be helpful to monitor quality of life using a questionnaire such as the AGHDA (adult GHD assessment) questionnaire.

GH therapy in special situations

- *Pregnancy* There are currently no data on GH replacement in pregnancy. There are occasional reports of continued GH replacement throughout pregnancy with no adverse effect.
- *Critical illness* There is no good evidence for a beneficial effect of GH replacement during critical illness. Patients should continue GH replacement during non-severe illness, but many endocrinologists would suggest that GH should be discontinued in patients who are severely ill: for example, receiving major surgery or on ITU.
- *Cardiac failure* GH treatment has recently been suggested as a potential therapy in dilated cardiomyopathy. Longer term data are required in this group of patients.

Adverse effects of GH replacement

- Sodium and water retention.
  - weight gain
  - carpal tunnel syndrome
- Hyperinsulinaemia.
- Arthralgia (possibly due to intra-articular cartilage swelling).
- Myalgia.
- Benign intracranial hypertension (resolves on stopping treatment).
- There are no data to suggest that GH therapy affects tumour development. (No evidence from long-term studies in children of increased risk of recurrence with GH treatment. Insufficient long-term data in adults.)

Contraindications to GH replacement

- active malignancy
- benign intracranial hypertension
- pre-proliferative/proliferative retinopathy in diabetes mellitus.

• As the long-term safety and efficacy of GH replacement in adults is as yet unknown, it is recommended that patients receiving GH therapy should remain under the care of an endocrinologist. There are large databases of patients receiving GH in order to monitor and determine these questions regarding long-term benefits and safety, particularly with regard to cardiovascular risk.

Further reading

Carroll PV, Christ ER, Bengtsson BA *et al.*, GH deficiency in adulthood and the effects of GH replacement: a review. *Journal of Clinical Endocrinology and Metabolism* 1998;83: 382–395.

Consensus Guidelines for the Diagnosis and Treatment of Adults with GH deficiency: Summary Statement of the GH Research Society Workshop on adult GH deficiency. *Journal of Clinical Endocrinology and Metabolism* 1998;83: 379–381.

Chapter 16
Pituitary tumours

Pathogenesis

The mechanism of pituitary tumourogenesis remains largely unclear. Pituitary adenomas are monoclonal, supporting the theory that there are intrinsic molecular events leading to pituitary tumourogenesis. However, the mutations (e.g. p53) found in other tumour types are only rarely found. A role for hormonal factors and in particular the hypothalamic hormones in tumour progression is likely.

Table 16.1 Approximate relative frequencies of pituitary tumours

Tumour type	Prevalence	Annual incidence
Incidental pituitary microadenomas	10–25% autopsies	
Clinically overt pituitary adenomas		1–2/100 000
Acromegaly	60 cases/million	4 cases/million
Cushing's syndrome		2 cases/million
Non-functioning adenoma		6 cases/million
Prolactinomas		10 cases/million (if hyperprolactinaemia is considered, then higher incidence)

NB Good epidemiological data are lacking except in acromegaly. Many of these figures derive from the pre-MRI era.

Molecular mechanisms of pituitary tumour pathogenesis

Activation of oncogenes

* *Gsα mutation* found in up to 40% GH-secreting tumours (less in non-Caucasians), and also described in a minority of NFAs and ACTH-secreting tumours.

* *Ras mutation* found in aggressive tumours and mainly pituitary carcinomas. ?Role in malignant transformation.

* *PTTG (pituitary tumour transforming gene)* has recently been described and found to be over-expressed in pituitary tumours. Its role in tumour pathogenesis is as yet uncertain.

Inactivation of tumour suppressor genes (TSG)

* *MEN-1 gene* LOH at 11q13 had been previously demonstrated in up to 20% sporadic pituitary tumours; however, the expression of the MEN-1 gene product, menin, is not down-regulated in the majority of sporadic pituitary tumours.

* *Rb gene* Mutations in mice lead to intermediate lobe corticotroph adenomas; however, no mutations have been demonstrated in human pituitary adenomas.

Cyclins and modulators of cyclin activity

* Mutations of the cyclin-dependent kinases *p27 and p18* are rare in human pituitary tumours (unlike studies in mice). p27 may be translationally down-regulated and p16 may be transcriptionally silenced by methylation of its gene. Cyclin D1 over-expression may be an early step in pituitary tumourogenesis as it is commonly found in different tumour types.

* *p53* Mutations are rare in pituitary tumours.

Alterations in receptor and growth factor expression (e.g. TGF, activin, bFGF)

No consistent patterns have emerged.

Further reading

Asa SL, Ezzat S. The cytogenesis and pathogenesis of pituitary adenomas. *Endocrine Reviews* 1998;19: 798–827.

Chapter 17
Prolactinomas

Epidemiology

- Prolactinomas are the commonest functioning pituitary tumour.
- Post-mortem studies show microprolactinomas in 10% the population.
- During life, microprolactinomas are commoner than macro-prolactinomas, and there is a female preponderance of micro-prolactinomas.

Pathogenesis

Unknown. Occur in 20% of patients with MEN-1. (Prolactinomas are commonest pituitary tumour in MEN-1 and may be more aggressive than sporadic prolactinomas.) Malignant prolactinomas are very rare and may harbour *ras* mutations.

Causes of hyperprolactinaemia

- *Physiological*
  - pregnancy
  - sexual intercourse
  - nipple stimulation/suckling
  - neonatal
  - stress
- *Pituitary tumour*
  - prolactinomas
  - mixed GH/PRL secreting tumour
  - macroadenoma compressing stalk
  - empty sella
- *Hypothalamic disease* mass compressing stalk (craniopharyngioma, meningioma, neurofibromatosis)
- *Infiltration* sarcoidosis, Langerhans cell histiocytosis
- *Stalk section* head injury, surgery
- *Cranial irradiation*
- *Drug treatment*
  - dopamine receptor antagonists (metoclopramide, domperidone)
  - neuroleptics* (thioridazine, chlorpromazine, haloperidol, sulpiride, fluphenazine, flupenthixol)
  - antidepressants (tricyclics, selective serotonin reuptake inhibitors, monoamine oxidase inhibitors)
  - cardiovascular drugs (verapamil, methyldopa)
  - opiates
  - protease inhibitors (e.g. ritonavir, indinavir, zidovudine)
  - others (bezafibrate, omeprazole, H2 antagonists)
- *Metabolic*
  - hypothyroidism (TRH increases PRL)
  - chronic renal failure (reduced PRL clearance)
  - severe liver disease (disordered hypothalamic regulation)
- *Other*
  - PCOS (can make differential diagnosis of menstrual problems difficult)
  - chest wall lesions – zoster, burns, trauma (stimulation of suckling reflex).

---

* clozapine, quetiapine and olanzapine are antipsychotics with little or no effect on prolactin.

Clinical features

Hyperprolactinaemia (microadenomas and macroadenomas)

* Galactorrhoea (up to 90% women, 10–20% men).

* Disturbed gonadal function in women presents with menstrual disturbance (up to 95%) – amenorrhoea, oligomenorrhoea, or with infertility, and reduced libido.

* Disturbed gonadal function in men presents with loss of libido and/or erectile dysfunction. Presentation with reduced fertility and oligospermia or gynaecomastia is unusual.

* Hyperprolactinaemia is associated with a long-term risk of reduced BMD.

* Hyperprolactinaemia inhibits GnRH release, leading to reduced LH secretion. There may be a direct action of PRL on the ovary to interfere with LH and FSH signalling which inhibits oestradiol and progesterone secretion and also follicle maturation.

Mass effects (macroadenomas only)

* Headaches and visual field defects (uni- or bitemporal field defects).

* Hypopituitarism.

* Invasion of the cavernous sinus may lead to cranial nerve palsies.

* Occasionally very invasive tumours may erode bone and present with a CSF leak or secondary meningitis.

Investigation

Serum PRL

* The differential diagnosis of elevated PRL is shown on p. 137. Note that the stress of venepuncture may cause mild hyperprolactinaemia, so 2–3 levels should be checked, preferably through an indwelling cannula after 30 min.
* Serum PRL >3000 mU/L is suggestive of a tumour – either a microprolactinoma or a macroadenoma compressing the pituitary stalk with loss of dopamine inhibitory tone to the lactotroph and subsequent hyperprolactinaemia.
* Serum PRL >6000 mU/L is diagnostic of a macroprolactinoma.
* Serum PRL 3000–6000 mU/L in association with a macroadenoma may be due to disconnection or due to a macroprolactinoma. Since the serum PRL falls with dopamine agonist treatment in either situation, but tumour shrinkage occurs only with macroprolactinomas, these patients should be carefully followed if treated with dopamine agonists and rescanned at 6 weeks. Lack of tumour shrinkage suggests a macroadenoma with stalk effect and surgery is advisable.
* *Hook effect* This occurs where the assay utilizes antibodies recognizing two ends of the molecule. One is used to capture the molecule, and one to label it. If PRL levels are very high, it may be bound by one antibody but not by the other. Thus above a certain concentration, the signal will reduce rather than increase and very high PRL levels will be spuriously reported as normal.

Thyroid function and renal function

Hypothyroidism and chronic renal failure are causes of hyperprolactinaemia.

Dynamic tests

These tests are used by some groups to attempt to differentiate between true idiopathic hyperprolactinaemia and hyperprolactinaemia due to an undetectable microprolactinoma.

Dopamine antagonist test

* I/v metoclopramide (10 mg).
* *Normal/hyperprolactinaemia due to other causes* At least twofold rise in PRL. No change in TSH.
* *Prolactinomas* Blunted PRL response and/or exaggerated TSH response

TRH test (p. 111)

* 200 μg TRH i/v
* Serum PRL at 0, 20 and 60 min.
* *Prolactinomas* blunted rise in PRL.

Imaging

* *MRI* Microadenomas usually appear as hypointense lesions within the pituitary on T1 weighted images. Negative imaging is an indication for contrast enhancement with gadolinium. Stalk deviation or gland asymmetry may also suggest microadenoma.

* Macroadenomas are space-occupying tumours often associated with bony erosion and/or cavernous sinus invasion

> **'Big' PRL**
>
> Occasionally, larger forms of PRL are detected in the circulation. Although these are measurable in the prolactin assay, they do not interfere with reproductive function. The most common is 'macroprolactin'. Typically there is hyperproctinaemia with regular ovulatory menstrual cycles. Assays for macroprolactin are available.

Hyperprolactinaemia and drugs

Antipsychotic agents are the most likely psychotropic agents to cause hyperprolactinaemia. If dose reduction is not possible or not effective, then an MRI to exclude a prolactinoma, and treatment of hypogonadism may be indicated. Where dopamine antagonism is the mechanism of action of the drug, then dopamine agonists may reduce efficacy. Drug-induced increases in PRL are usually <5000 mU/L.

'Idiopathic' hyperprolactinaemia

When no cause is found following evaluation as above, the hyperprolactinaemia is designated idiopathic, but in many cases is likely to be due to a tiny microprolactinoma which is not demonstrable on current imaging techniques. In other cases it may be due to alterations in hypothalamic regulation. Follow-up of these patients shows that in 1/3, PRL levels return to normal, in 10–15% there is a further increase in PRL, and in the remainder PRL levels remain stable.

Treatment

Aims of therapy

- *Microprolactinomas* restoration of gonadal function.
- *Macroprolactinomas*
  - reduction in tumour size and prevention of tumour expansion
  - restoration of gonadal function.
- Although microprolactinomas may expand in size without treatment, the majority do not (<7%). Therefore although restoration of gonadal function is usually achieved by lowering PRL levels. Ensuring adequate sex hormone replacement is an alternative if the tumour is monitored in size.
- Macroprolactinomas, however, will continue to expand and lead to pressure effects. Definitive treatment of the tumour is therefore necessary.

Drug therapy – dopamine agonists

- Dopamine agonist treatment (see p. 224) leads to suppression of PRL in most patients, with secondary effects of normalization of gonadal function and termination of galactorrhoea. Tumour shrinkage occurs at a variable rate and extent, and must be carefully monitored.
- *Cabergoline* is more effective in normalization of PRL in microprolactinoma (83% compared with 59% on bromocriptine) with fewer side-effects than *bromocriptine*.
- In patients with macroadenomas and PRL 3000–5000 mU/L a trial of dopamine agonist therapy is reasonable provided that surgical intervention occurs if there is visual deterioration or failure to shrink significantly at 6–12 weeks. Approximately 60% of patients will show normalization of PRL and tumour shrinkage with bromocriptine or cabergoline.
- Dopamine agonist resistance may occur when there are reduced numbers of D2 receptors.

Surgery (see p. 212)

- Since the introduction of dopamine agonist treatment, transsphenoidal surgery is indicated only for patients who are resistant to or intolerant of dopamine agonist treatment. The cure rate for macroprolactinomas treated with surgery is poor (30%), and therefore drug treatment is first-line in tumours of all size. Occasionally surgery may be required for patients with CSF leak secondary to an invasive macroprolactinoma. Cure rates for microprolactinomas treated with surgery are >80%, but the risk of hypopituitarism (GH deficient in 25%) and recurrence (4% at 5 yrs) makes this a second-line option.

- The surgical management of a CSF leak can be very difficult in patients with very invasive tumours. Tumour shrinkage with dopamine agonists will either precipitate or worsen the leak, with the subsequent risk of meningitis. There is no evidence for the long-term use of prophylactic antibiotics in this group, but patients at risk should be informed of the warning symptoms and advised to seek expert medical attention urgently.

Radiotherapy (see p. 218)

- Standard pituitary irradiation leads to slow reduction (over years) of PRL in the majority of patients. While waiting for radiotherapy to be effective, dopamine agonist therapy is continued, but should be withdrawn on a biannual basis at least to assess if it is still required.

- Radiotherapy is rarely indicated in the management of patients with microprolactinomas. It is useful in the treatment of macro-prolactinomas once the tumour has been shrunk away from the chiasm.

Prognosis

- The natural history of microprolactinomas is difficult to assess. However, they are a common post-mortem incidental finding, and <17% show any increase in tumour size. It has been demonstrated that hyperprolactinaemia in approximately 1/3 of women will resolve particularly after the menopause or pregnancy. This shows that patients receiving dopamine agonist treatment for micropro-lactinoma should have treatment withdrawn intermittently to assess the continued requirement for it, and certainly the dose may be titrated downwards over time.

- There are few data on dopamine agonist withdrawal in macro-prolactinomas in the absence of definitive treatment (radiotherapy or surgery). There are data suggesting that cautious attempts at dose reduction could be considered after 2–5 years. These patients would need close monitoring and scans. In the absence of definitive management of the tumour, complete withdrawal of drug treatment is likely to be associated with tumour enlargement.

Management of prolactinomas in pregnancy

See p. 512.

Further reading

Bevan JS, Webster J, Burke CW, Scanlon MF. Dopamine agonists and pituitary tumour shrinkage. *Endocrinology Reviews* 1992; 13: 220–240.

Molitch ME. Pregnancy and the hyperprolactinaemic woman. *New England Journal of Medicine* 1985; 312: 1364–1370.

Molitch ME. Pathologic hyperprolactinaemia. *Endocrinology and Metabolism Clinics of North America* 1992; 21: 877–910.

Tsagarakis S, Grossman A, Plowman PN, Jones AE, Touzel R, Rees LH, Wass JAH, Besser GM. Megavoltage pituitary irradiation in the management of prolactinomas: long-term follow-up. *Clinical Endocrinology* 1991; 34: 399–406.

Chapter 18
Acromegaly

Definition

Acromegaly is the clinical condition resulting from prolonged excessive GH and hence, IGF-1 secretion in adults. GH secretion is characterized by blunting of pulsatile secretion and failure of GH to become undetectable during the 24 h day, unlike normal controls.

Epidemiology

• Rare. Equal sex distribution.

• Prevalence 40–60 cases/million population. Annual incidence of new cases in the UK is 4/million population.

• Onset is insidious, and there is therefore often a considerable delay between onset of clinical features and diagnosis. Most cases are diagnosed at 40–60 years. Typically acromegaly occurring in an older patient is a milder disease with lower GH levels and a smaller tumour.

Pituitary gigantism

The clinical syndrome resulting from excess GH secretion in children prior to fusion of the epiphyses.

• Rare.

• Increased growth velocity without premature pubertal manifestations should arouse suspicion of pituitary gigantism.

• *Differential diagnosis* Marfan's syndrome, neurofibromatosis, pubertal disorders, cerebral gigantism (large at birth with accelerated linear growth, and disproportionately large extremities – associated normal IGF-1 and GH).

• Arm span > standing height is compatible with eunochoid features, and suggests onset of disease before epiphyseal fusion (pituitary gigantism).

Causes

- *Pituitary adenoma* (>99% of cases) Macroadenomas > micro-adenomas. Local invasion is common, but frank carcinomas are very rare.
- *GHRH secretion*
  - hypothalamic secretion
  - ectopic GHRH e.g. carcinoid tumour (pancreas, lung) or other neuroendocrine tumours
- *Ectopic GH secretion* Very rare. One report of a pancreatic islet cell tumour secreting GH and one of a lymphoreticulosis.
- There has been some progress on the molecular pathogenesis of the GH secreting pituitary adenomas – as mutations of the Gsα are found in up to 40% of tumours. This leads to an abnormality of the G protein that usually inhibits GTPase activity in the somatotroph.

Associations

- *MEN-1* less common than prolactinomas (p. 718).
- *Carney complex* AD, spotty cutaneous pigmentation, cardiac and other myxomas, and endocrine overactivity, particularly Cushing's syndrome due to nodular adrenal cortical hyperplasia and GH secreting pituitary tumours in less than 10% of cases. Mainly due to activating mutations of protein kinase A (p. 732).
- *Isolated familial somatotrophinomas* existence of two or more cases of acromegaly or gigantism in a family that does not exhibit MEN-1 or Carney complex. (Possibly linked to chromosome 11q13.)

Clinical features

The clinical features arise from the effects of excess GH/IGF-1, excess PRL in some (as there is co-secretion of PRL in a minority (30%) of tumours, or rarely stalk compression), and the tumour mass.

Symptoms
- increased sweating (>80% of patients)
- headaches (independent of tumour effect)
- tiredness and lethargy
- joint pains
- change in ring or shoe size.

Signs
- *Facial appearance* Coarse features, oily skin, frontal bossing, enlarged nose, deep nasolabial furrows, prognathism and increased interdental separation.
- *Deep voice* (laryngeal thickening).
- *Tongue enlargement* (macroglossia).
- *Musculoskeletal changes* enlargement of hands and feet, degenerative changes in joints lead to osteoarthritis. Generalized myopathy.
- *Soft tissue swelling* may lead to entrapment neuropathies such as carpal tunnel syndrome (40% of patients).
- *Goitre and other organomegaly* (liver, heart, kidney).

Complications
- hypertension (40%)
- insulin resistance and impaired glucose tolerance (40%)/ diabetes mellitus (20%)
- obstructive sleep apnoea (due to soft tissue swelling in nasopharyngeal region)
- increased risk of colonic polyps and colonic carcinoma (extent currently considered controversial)
- ischaemic heart disease and cerebrovascular disease
- congestive cardiac failure.

Effects of tumour
- visual field defects
- hypopituitarism.

Investigations

Oral glucose tolerance test

- In acromegaly, there is failure to suppress GH to <2 mU/L in response to a 75 g oral glucose load. In contrast, the normal response is GH suppression to undetectable levels.
- *False positives* chronic renal and liver failure, malnutrition, diabetes mellitus, heroin addiction, adolescence (due to high pubertal GH surges).

Random GH

Not useful in the diagnosis of acromegaly as although normal healthy subjects have undetectable GH levels throughout the day, there are pulses of GH which are impossible to differentiate from the levels seen in acromegaly. However, a random GH <1 mU/L excludes the diagnosis.

IGF-1

Useful in addition to the OGTT in differentiating patients with acromegaly from normals, as it is almost invariably elevated in acromegaly except in severe intercurrent illness. It has a long half-life as it is bound to binding proteins, and reflects the effect of GH on tissues. However, abnormalities of GH secretion may remain while IGF-1 is normal.

IGFBP3

IGFBP3 concentrations correlate with IGF-1, and the use of this assay in both the diagnosis and monitoring of acromegaly has been advocated. It does not give such clear differentiation in the diagnosis as IGF.

TRH test (p. 111)

The normal GH response at 20 and 60 min following 200 g TRH i/v is GH suppression; however, 80% of patients with acromegaly show an increase (by 50% of basal). This test is usually not required as the OGTT and IGF-1 usually provide the diagnosis. It may be helpful in patients with equivocal results.

MRI

MRI usually demonstrates the tumour, and whether there is extra-sellar extension either suprasellar or into the cavernous sinus. In addition, plain radiographs may demonstrate enlargement of the pituitary fossa and frontal sinuses, although these are usually not performed routinely.

Pituitary function testing (see p. 104)

Serum PRL should be measured as some tumours co-secrete both GH and PRL.

Serum calcium

Some patients are hypercalcaemic due to increased 1,25-DHCC as GH stimulates renal 1α-hydroxylase. There may be an increased likelihood of renal stones due to hypercalcaemia as well as hypercalciuria (which occurs in 80%). Rarely hypercalcaemia may be due to associated MEN-1 and hyperparathyroidism.

GHRH

Occasionally it is not possible to demonstrate a pituitary tumour, or pituitary histology reveals hyperplasia. A serum GHRH in addition to radiology of the chest and abdomen may then be indicated to identify the cause, usually a GHRH carcinoid of lung or pancreas.

GHDC

- GH taken at 4–5 time points during the day.
- This is used to assess response to treatment following surgery or radiotherapy, and also to assess GH suppression on somatostatin analogues, in order to determine whether an increase in dose is required.
- It does not have a role in the diagnosis of acromegaly, but in acromegaly GH is detectable in all samples in contrast to normal. The degree of elevation of GH is relevant to the response to all forms of treatment; the higher the GH the less frequent is treatment by surgery, drugs, or radiotherapy effective.

Differential diagnosis of elevated GH

* pain
* pregnancy
* puberty
* adolescence if tall
* stress
* chronic renal failure
* chronic liver failure
* heart failure
* diabetes mellitus
* malnutrition
* prolonged fast.
* severe illness
* heroin addiction

Note on units for GH assay

* GH concentrations may be measured in mU/L or µg/L. The equivalent ratio of mU/L to µg/L was previously considered to be 2 and now 3.
* To improve standardization, it is recommended that the GH reference preparation should be a recombinant 22 kDa hGH; presently 88/624.
* There is currently no acceptable IGF-1 reference preparation.

Management

The management strategy depends on the individual patient, and also on the tumour size. A tumour causing compressive effects requires definitive management, whereas microadenomas do not necessarily need tumour removal. Lowering of GH is essential in all situations.

Trans-sphenoidal surgery (see p. 212)

* This is usually the first line for treatment in most centres.
* Reported cure rates vary: 40–91% for microadenomas and 10–48% for macroadenomas, depending on surgical expertise.
* A GHDC should be performed following surgery to assess whether 'safe' levels of GH and IGF-1 have been attained. If the mean GH is < 5 mU/L then the patient can be followed up with annual IGF-1 and/or GH assessment. If safe levels of GH have not been achieved, then medical treatment and or radiotherapy is indicated.

Role of preoperative octreotide treatment

This leads to some tumour shrinkage in at least 40% of cases, and it has been suggested that it may lead to reduced operative morbidity, and possibly improve surgical results.

Tumour recurrence following surgery

This is defined as tumour regrowth and increase in GH levels leading to active acromegaly following postoperative normalization of GH levels. Using the definition of postoperative cure as mean GH <5 mU/L, the reported recurrence rate is low (6% at 5 years).

Radiotherapy (see p. 218)

* This is usually reserved for patients following unsuccessful trans-sphenoidal surgery, only occasionally is it used as primary therapy. The largest fall in GH occurs during the first 2 years, but GH continues to fall after this. However, normalization of mean GH may take several years and during this time adjunctive medical treatment (usually with somatostatin analogues) is required. With a starting mean GH >50 mU/L, it takes on average 6 years to achieve mean GH <5 mU/L compared with 4 years with starting mean GH <50 mU/L.
* After radiotherapy, somatostatin analogues should be withdrawn on an annual basis to perform a GHDC to assess progress and identify when mean GH <5 mU/L and therefore radiotherapy has been effective and somatostatin analogue treatment is no longer required.

Definition of cure

◆ Epidemiological data suggest that a mean GH <5 mU/L should be the aim of treatment, as this is associated with reduction of the increased mortality associated with acromegaly to that of the normal population. More recently normalization of IGF-1 has also been shown in one study to be associated with reduction of increased mortality to normal.

◆ For this reason, patients are monitored during treatment using a GH day curve aiming for a mean of <5 mU/L over 5 points throughout the day. Others use suppression to <2 mU/L on an OGTT as this has been shown to correlate well with mean GH. It is likely that normalization of IGF-1 may also be used, but there are limited epidemiological data on this approach.

Colonic polyps and acromegaly

◆ Increased incidence of *colonic polyps and colonic carcinoma* has been reported by many groups. Both retrospective and prospective studies have demonstrated that 9–39% of acromegalic patients studied have colonic polyps and 0–20% have been shown to have colonic carcinoma.

◆ *Mechanism* IGF-1 and/or GH are implicated as both may stimulate colonic mucosal turnover. However, some studies have failed to demonstrate a direct relationship between serum levels and polyps/carcinoma.

◆ *Importance* Patients with acromegaly are at increased risk and therefore need screening for polyps. It has been proposed that all patients aged >40 years should have 3 yearly routine colonoscopy, and those with polyps should receive annual colonoscopy. Agreement has not been reached on the frequency of follow up colonoscopy.

Drug treatment

Somatostatin analogues (see p. 226)

- Somatostatin analogues lead to suppression of GH secretion in 60% of patients with acromegaly. At least 40% of patients are complete responders and somatostatin analogues will lead to normalization of mGH (<5 mU/L) and IGF-1. However, some patients are partial responders and although somatostatin analogues will lead to lowering of mean GH, they do not suppress to normal despite dose escalation.

- Acute response to these drugs is assessed by measuring GH at hourly intervals for 6 h following the injection of 50–100 μg octreotide s/c. This predicts long-term response.

- The usual dose required is 50–200 μg s/c 3xdaily. More recently the depot preparations lanreotide SR, lanreotide autogel, and octreotide LR have become available. Lanreotide SR is administered at 30 mg i/m every 14 days with dose escalations up to every 7 days if adequate GH suppression does not occur. Octreotide LAR 20 mg i/m is administered every 4 weeks, with dose alterations either down or up to 10–30 mg every 3 months. Lanreotide autogel 90 μg i/m is administered every 4 weeks with dose alteration either down to 60 mg or up to 120 mg every 3 months.

- These drugs may be used as primary therapy where the tumour does not cause mass effects, or in patients who have received surgery and or radiotherapy who have elevated mean GH.

Dopamine agonists (see p. 224)

These drugs do lead to lowering of GH levels, but very rarely lead to normalization of mGH or IGF-1 (<10%). They may be helpful particularly if there is coexistent secretion of PRL, and in these cases there may be significant tumour shrinkage. Cabergoline has recently been shown to be more effective than bromocriptine and may lead to IGF-1 normalization in up to 30%. Doses of 10–60 mg bromocriptine daily or cabergoline 1.5–3 mg weekly are used.

GH receptor antagonists (pegvisomant)

A new GH receptor antagonist has been developed and early data suggest normalization of IGF-1 in more than 90% of patients. More data on the effect on tumour size are required.

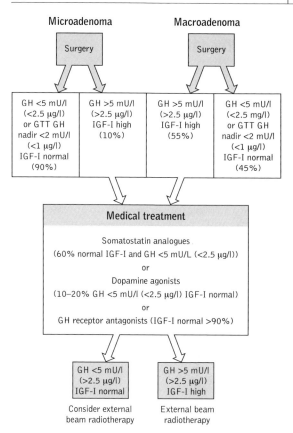

Fig. 18.1 Treatment paradigms in acromegaly. Reproduced with permission of BioScientifica Ltd.

Mortality data

- Mortality in untreated patients is double that of the normal population.
- Major causes include cardiovascular, cerebrovascular, and respiratory disease. More effective treatment has now increased life expectancy and the true risk of malignancy in this group will become clearer.

Further reading

Bates AS, Van't Hoff W, Jones JM, Clayton RN. An audit of outcome of treatment in acromegaly. *Quarterly Journal of Medicine* 1993;86: 293–299.

Jenkins PJ, Fairclough PD, Richards T, Lowe DG, Monson J, Grossman A, Wass JAH, Besser M. Acromegaly, colonic polyps and carcinoma. *Clinical Endocrinology* 1997;47: 17–22.

Orme SM, McNally RJQ, Cartwright RA, Belcheltz PE. Mortality and Cancer Incidence in Acromegaly: A retrospective cohort study JCEM 1998; 83: 2730–2734.

Wass JAH (ed.) Handbook of Acromegaly (2001). BioScientifica, Bristol.

Chapter 19
Cushing's disease

Definition

Cushing's syndrome is an illness resulting from excess cortisol secretion which has a high mortality if left untreated. There are several causes of hypercortisolaemia which must be differentiated, and the commonest cause is iatrogenic (inhaled or topical steroids). It is important to decide whether the patient has true Cushing's syndrome rather than pseudo-Cushing's associated with depression or alcoholism. Secondly, ACTH-dependent Cushing's must be differentiated from ACTH-independent disease (usually due to an adrenal adenoma or rarely carcinoma – see page 290). Once a diagnosis of ACTH-dependent disease has been established, it is important to differentiate between pituitary dependent (Cushing's disease) and ectopic secretion (see page 774).

Epidemiology of Cushing's disease

- rare, annual incidence approximately 2/million.
- commoner in women (3–15 : 1, F : M).
- age – most commonly 20–40 years.

Pathophysiology

- The vast majority of Cushing's syndrome is due to a pituitary ACTH-secreting corticotroph microadenoma. The underlying aetiology is ill-understood.
- Occasionally corticotroph adenomas reach larger sizes (macroadenomas) and rarely become invasive or malignant. The tumours typically maintain some responsiveness to the usual feedback control factors that influence the normal corticotoph (e.g. high doses of glucocorticoids, and CRH). However, this may be lost and the tumours become fully autonomous, particularly in Nelson's syndrome.
- NB Crooke's hyaline change is a fibrillary appearance seen in the non-tumorous corticotroph associated with elevated cortisol levels from any cause.

Causes of Cushing's syndrome

- pseudo-Cushing's syndrome
  - alcoholism   <1%
  - severe depression   1%
- ACTH-dependent
  - pituitary adenoma   68% (Cushing's disease)
  - ectopic ACTH syndrome   12%
  - ectopic CRH secretion   <1%
- ACTH-independent
  - adrenal adenoma   10%
  - adrenal carcinoma   8%
  - nodular hyperplasia   1%

Clinical features

See facing page.

The features of Cushing's syndrome are progressive and may be present for several years prior to diagnosis. A particular difficulty may occur in a patients with cyclical Cushing's, where the features and biochemical manifestations appear and disappear with a variable periodicity.

Clinical features

* *Facial appearance* round plethoric complexion, acne and hirsutism, thinning of scalp hair
* *Weight gain* truncal obesity, buffalo hump, supraclavicular fat pads.
* *Skin* thin and fragile due to loss of s/c tissue, purple striae on abdomen, breasts, thighs, axillae (in contrast to silver healed postpartum striae), easy bruising, tinea versicolor, occasionally pigmentation due to ACTH.
* Proximal *muscle weakness*.
* *Mood disturbance* labile, depression, insomnia, psychosis.
* *Menstrual disturbance.*
* *Low libido and impotence.*
* *Growth arrest* in children.

Associated features

* Hypertension (>50%) due to mineralocorticoid effects of cortisol. (Cortisol overwhelms the renal 11β-hydroxysteroid dehydrogenase enzyme protecting the mineralocorticoid receptor from cortisol). Cortisol may also increase angiotensinogen levels.
* Impaired glucose tolerance/diabetes mellitus (30%).
* Osteopenia and osteoporosis (leading to fractures of spine and ribs).
* Vascular disease.
* Susceptibility to infections.

Investigation

Does the patient have Cushing's syndrome?

Outpatient tests

- *24 h urinary free cortisol* This test can be useful for outpatient screening – however the false negative rate of 5–10% means that it should not be used alone.

- *Overnight dexamethasone suppression test* Administration of 1 mg dexamethasone at midnight is followed by a serum cortisol measurement at 9 a.m. The false negative value is 2% of normal individuals but rises to <20% in obese or hospitalized patients.

- If both the above tests are normal, Cushing's syndrome is unlikely.

Inpatient tests

- *Midnight cortisol* Loss of circadian rhythm of cortisol secretion is seen in Cushing's syndrome and this is demonstrated by measuring a serum cortisol at midnight (patient must be asleep for this test to be valid). In normal subjects the cortisol at this time is at a nadir (<50 nmol/L), but in patients with Cushing's syndrome it is elevated.

- *Low dose dexamethasone suppression test* Administration of 0.5 mg dexamethasone 6 hourly for 48 h at 9 a.m., 3 p.m., 9 p.m. and 3 a.m. should lead to complete suppression of cortisol to <50 nmol/L in normal subjects. Serum cortisol is measured at time 0 and 48 h (day 2).

- NB Oestrogen effect on CBG. False positive results may also occur if dexamethasone metabolism is increased by drugs that induce liver enzyme activity such as rifampicin and phenytoin.

- Patients with pseudo-Cushing's syndrome will also show loss of diurnal rhythm and lack of low dose suppressibility. However, alcoholics return to normal cortisol secretory dynamics after a few days' abstinence in hospital. Severe depression can be more difficult to differentiate, particularly since this may be a feature of Cushing's syndrome itself. Typically patients with pseudo-Cushing's show a normal cortisol rise with hypoglycaemia (tested using insulin tolerance test), whereas patients with true Cushing's syndrome show a blunted rise. However, this is not 100% reliable, as up to 20% of patients with Cushing's syndrome (especially those with cyclical disease) show a normal cortisol rise with hypoglycaemia.

Cyclical Cushing's

A small group of patients with Cushing's syndrome have alternating normal and abnormal cortisol levels on an irregular basis. All causes of Cushing's syndrome may be associated with cyclical secretion of cortisol. Clearly the results of dynamic testing can only be interpreted when the disease is shown to be active (elevated urinary cortisol secretion and loss of normal circadian rhythm and suppressability on dexamethasone).

Table 19.1 Screening tests for Cushing's syndrome

Test	False positives	False negatives	Sensitivity
24 h urinary free cortisol	1%	5–10%	95%
Overnight 1 mg dexamethasone suppression test	2% normal 13% obese 23% hospital inpatients	2%	
Midnight cortisol	?	0	100%
Low-dose dexamethasone suppression test	<2%	2%	98%

What is the underlying cause?

ACTH

- Once the presence of Cushing's syndrome has been confirmed, a serum basal ACTH should be measured to differentiate between ACTH dependent and ACTH independent aetiologies (Fig. 19.1).

- The basal ACTH is, however, of very little value in differentiating between pituitary dependent Cushing's syndrome and ectopic Cushing's syndrome as there is considerable overlap between the two groups although patients with ectopic disease tend to have higher ACTH levels (Fig. 19.1).

Serum potassium

A rapidly spun potassium is a useful discriminatory test as hypokalaemia <3.2 mmol/L is found in almost 100% of patients with ectopic secretion of ACTH but less than 10% of patients with pituitary dependent disease.

High dose dexamethasone suppression test

The high dose dexamethasone suppression test is performed in an identical way to the low dose test but with 2 mg doses of dexamethasone. In Cushing's disease the cortisol falls by >50% of the basal value. In ectopic disease, there is no suppression. However, approximately 10% of cases of ectopic disease – particularly those due to carcinoid tumours show >50% suppression, and 10% of patients with Cushing's disease do not suppress.

Corticotrophin releasing hormone test (Fig. 19.2)

- The administration of 100 μg of CRH i/v leads to an exaggerated rise in cortisol and ACTH in 95% of patients with pituitary-dependent Cushing's syndrome. There are occasional reports of patients with ectopic disease who show a similar response.

- Because of the spontaneous fluctuation of cortisol levels in patients with Cushing's syndrome – a response to CRH is defined as a rise in peak cortisol of 20% above basal and of 50% in ACTH.

Inferior petrosal sinus sampling (Fig. 19.3)

- Bilateral simultaneous inferior petrosal sinus sampling with measurement of ACTH centrally and in the periphery in the basal state and following stimulation with intravenous CRH (100 μg) allows differentiation between pituitary dependent and ectopic disease. A central to peripheral ratio of >2 prior to CRH is very suggestive of pituitary dependent disease, and >3 following CRH gives a diagnostic accuracy of approaching 100% for pituitary dependent disease.

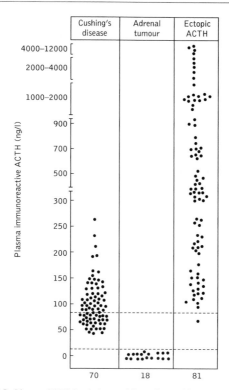

Fig. 19.1 Plasma ACTH levels (9 a.m.) in patients with pituitary dependent Cushing's disease, adrenal tumours and ectopic ACTH secretion. © Reprinted from Besser & Thorner *Clinical endocrinology*, by permission of the publisher Mosby.

Table 19.2 Investigation of ACTH-dependent Cushing's syndrome

Test	Pituitary dependent disease (% with this finding)	Ectopic disease (% with this finding)
Serum potassium <3.2 mmol/L	10	100
Suppression of basal cortisol to over 50% on high dose dexamethasone suppression test	90	10
Exaggerated rise in cortisol on CRH test	95	<1

• The accurate lateralization of a tumour using the results from inferior petrosal sinus sampling (IPSS) is difficult as differences in blood flow and catheter placement, etc. will affect the results.

Pituitary imaging

MRI following gadolinium enhancement localizes corticotroph adenomas in up to 80% of cases. However, it should be remembered that at least 10% of the normal population harbour microadenomas and therefore the biochemical investigation of these patients is essential as a patient with an ectopic source to Cushing's syndrome may have a pituitary 'incidentaloma'.

Other pituitary function

Hypercortisolism suppresses the thyroidal, gonadal, and GH axes leading to lowered levels of TSH and thyroid hormones as well as reduced gonadotrophins, gonadal steroids and GH.

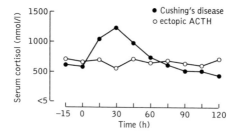

Fig. 19.2 CRH test in pituitary-dependent and ectopic disease. In the patient with pituitary-dependent disease, the characteristic marked plasma cortisol rise after an i/v bolus of 100 µg of CRH is seen. Serum cortisol levels are unaltered in the patient with ectopic ACTH secretion. © Reprinted from Besser & Thorner *Clinical endocrinology*, by permission of the publisher Mosby.

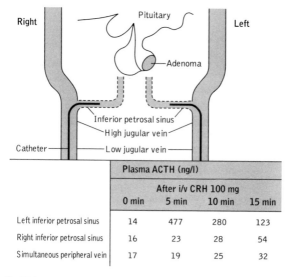

	Plasma ACTH (ng/l)			
	After i/v CRH 100 mg			
	0 min	5 min	10 min	15 min
Left inferior petrosal sinus	14	477	280	123
Right inferior petrosal sinus	16	23	28	54
Simultaneous peripheral vein	17	19	25	32

Fig. 19.3 Simultaneous bilateral inferior petrosal sinus and peripheral vein sampling for ACTH. The ratio of >3 between the left central and peripheral vein confirm a diagnosis of Cushing' disease. © Reprinted from Besser & Thorner *Clinical endocrinology*, by permission of the publisher Mosby.

Treatment

Trans-sphenoidal surgery (see p. 212)

- This is the first line option in most cases. Selective adenomectomy gives the greatest chance of cure with a reported remission rate of up to 90%. However, strict criteria of a postoperative cortisol of <50 nmol/L lead to lower cure rates, but much lower recurrence rates (<10% compared with up to 50% in those with detectable postoperative cortisols). This should be the current definition of successful surgery as the long-term outcome is significantly better in this group of patients.

- Complications of surgery may be higher in these patients as their preoperative general status and the condition of the tissues is poorer than other patients who are referred for surgery. It is often useful to administer medical treatment for at least 6 weeks prior to surgery to allow improvement in wound healing and reduce anaesthetic risk in those with severe metabolic problems.

Pituitary radiotherapy (see p. 218)

This is usually administered as second-line treatment following unsuccessful trans-sphenoidal surgery. As control of cortisol levels may take months to years, medical treatment to control cortisol levels while waiting for cortisol levels to fall is essential. A more rapid response to radiotherapy is seen in childhood.

Adrenalectomy

- This used to be the favoured form of treatment. It successfully controls cortisol hypersecretion in the majority of patients. Occasionally a remnant is left and leads to recurrent hypercortisolaemia.

- Nelson's syndrome may occur in up to 30% of patients. The administration of prophylactic radiotherapy reduces the liklihood of this complication. Careful follow-up of these patients is therefore essential to allow prompt treatment of the tumour. These tumours are associated with marked increase in ACTH, and associated pigmentation is common. Loss of normal responsiveness to glucocorticoids is characteristic and therefore biochemical monitoring should be performed at least annually by measuring a basal ACTH and re-checking it 1 and 2 h after the morning dose of glucocorticoid (ACTH curve).

Peri- and postoperative management following trans-sphenoidal surgery for Cushing's disease

• Perioperative hydrocortisone replacement is given in the standard way as it is assumed that the patient will become cortisol deficient after successful removal of the tumour.

• After 3–4 days, the evening steroid replacement is omitted, and 9 a.m. cortisol and ACTH checked the following day, and 24 h later after withholding steroids. Undetectable cortisol (<50 nmol/L) is suggestive of cure and glucocorticoid replacement is commenced. Cortisol 50–300 nmol/L is compatible with resolution of symptoms and a day curve should be performed. Patients with levels higher than 300 nmol/L should be considered for re-exploration and/or radiotherapy.

Nelson's syndrome

• Occurs in patients with Cushing's disease following adrenalectomy.

• Hyperpigmentation and an enlarging (often invasive) pituitary tumour associated with markedly elevated ACTH levels.

• Usually within 2 years of adrenalectomy.

- Bilateral adrenalectomy may still be indicated when pituitary surgery, radiotherapy and medical treatment have failed to control the disease. It is also helpful in Cushing's syndrome due to ectopic disease, when the ectopic source remains elusive or inoperable. Laparoscopic surgery minimalizes morbidity and complications.

Medical treatment

- This is indicated during the preoperative preparation of patients, or while awaiting radiotherapy to be effective or if surgery or radiotherapy are contra-indicated. *Metyrapone* is usually used first line, but *ketoconazole* should be used as first line in children as it is unassociated with increased adrenal metabolites. There is also a suggestion that ketoconazole may have a direct action on the corticotroph as well as lowering cortisol secretion.

- The dose of these drugs needs to be titrated against the cortisol results from a day curve (cortisol taken at 9 a.m., 12 noon, 3 p.m., 6 p.m.) aiming for a mean cortisol of 150–300 nmol/L as this approximates the normal production rate.

- Successful treatment (surgery or radiotherapy) of Cushing's disease leads to cortisol deficiency, and therefore glucocorticoid replacement therapy is essential. In addition patients who have undergone bilateral adrenalectomy require fludrocortisone. These patients should all receive instructions for intercurrent illness and carry a Medic-Alert bracelet and steroid card.

Table 19.3 Drug treatment of Cushing's syndrome

Drug	Dose	Action	Side-effects
Metyrapone	1–4 g/d (usually given in 4 divided doses)	11ß-hydroxylase inhibitor	Nausea Increased androgenic and mineralocorticoid precursors lead to hirsutism and hypertension
Ketoconazole	200–400 mg tds First line in children NB Avoid if taking H2 antagonists as acid required to metabolize active compound.	Direct inhibitor of P450 enzymes at several different sites	Abnormalities of liver function (usually reversible) Gynaecomastia
Mitotane (o-p- DDD)	4–12 g/d (begin at 0.5–1 g/d and gradually increase dose)	Inhibits steroidogenesis at the side-chain cleavage, 11 and 18-hydroxylase and 3ß-hydroxysteroid dehydrogenase Adrenolytic	Nausea and vomiting Cerebellar disturbance Somnolence Hypercholesterolaemia NB May increase clearance of steroids – replacement dosage may need to be increased NB May be teratogenic. Avoid if fertility desired.
Etomidate	Useful when parenteral treatment is required.	Inhibits side-chain cleavage and 11ß-hydroxylase.	

Definition of cure

Successful treatment for Cushing's disease leads to a cortisol that is undetectable (<50 nmol/L) following surgery. (This is due to the total suppression of cortisol production from the normal corticotroph in Cushing's disease). An undetectable postoperative cortisol leads to a significantly higher chance of long-term cure compared to the patients who had postoperative cortisols between 50 and 300 nmol/L.

Follow-up

- The aim of follow-up is
  - to detect recurrent Cushing's, and also
  - to recognize when recovery of the pituitary adrenal axis occurs.
- Therefore patients need to have regular assessment of cortisol production off glucocorticoid replacement. When cortisol is detectable following surgery, recurrent disease must be excluded (UFC and low dose dexamethasone suppression). If recurrence is excluded, it is then important to document the adequacy of the stress response once weaned off glucocorticoid replacement (insulin tolerance test).

Cushing's syndrome in children

In a series of 59 patients aged 4–20 years:

Causes

* pituitary dependent disease   85%
* adrenal disease   10%
* ectopic ACTH secretion   5%.

Initial presentation

* excessive weight gain   90%
* growth retardation   83%.

Below the age of 5 years, adrenal causes are common. In neonates and young children the McCune–Albright syndrome should be considered, whereas in late childhood and early adolescence, ACTH independence may suggest Carney's syndrome.

Treatment

* Trans-sphenoidal surgery is used as first line therapy in pituitary dependent Cushing's in children as in adults and is usually successful. Radiotherapy cures up to 85% children and this may be considered first line in some patients. Ketoconazole is the preferred medical therapy in this age group as it is not associated with increased adrenal androgens.

* The long-term management of children with Cushing's syndrome requires careful attention to growth as growth failure is a very common presentation of this condition. Postoperatively or after radiotherapy, GH therapy may restore growth and final height to normal.

Prognosis

- Untreated disease leads to an approximately 30–50% mortality at 5 years owing to vascular disease and increased susceptibility to infections.

- Treated Cushing's syndrome has a good prognosis. Patients who have an undetectable postoperative cortisol are very unlikely to recur (0–20%), whereas 50–75% recur if the postoperative cortisol is detectable.

- Although the physical features and severe psychological disorders associated with Cushing's improve or resolve within weeks or months of successful treatment, more subtle mood disturbance may persist for longer. In addition, it is likely that there is an increased cardiovascular risk.

- Osteoporosis will usually resolve in children, but may not improve significantly in older patients. Bone mineral density therefore requires monitoring and may need specific treatment. *Alendronate* has been shown to be effective therapy leading to improved bone mineral density in patients with Cushing's syndrome and osteoporosis. Hypertension has been shown to resolve in 80% and diabetes mellitus in up to 70%.

Further reading

Estrada J, Boronat M, Mielgo M, Magallon R, Millan I, Diez S, Lucas T, Barcelo B. The long-term outcome of pituitary irradiation after unsuccessful transsphenoidal surgery in Cushing's syndrome. *New England Journal of Medicine* 1997; 336: 172–177.

Howlett TA, Drury PL, Perry L, Doniach I, Rees LH, Besser GM. Diagnosis and management of ACTH-dependent Cushing's syndrome: comparison of the features in ectopic and pituitary ACTH production. *Clinical Endocrinology* 1986; 24: 699–713.

Magiakou MA, Mastorakos G, Oldfield EH, Gomez MT, Doppman JL, Cutler GB, Niemann LK, Chrousos GP. Cushing's syndrome in children and adolescents. *New England Journal of Medicine* 1994; 331: 629–636.

Newell-Price J, Trainer P, Besser M, Grossman A. The diagnosis and differential diagnosis of Cushing's syndrome and pseudo-Cushing's states. *Endocrinology Reviews* 1998; 19(5): 647–672.

Oldfield EH, Doppman JL, Nieman LK, Chrousos GP, Miller DL, Katz DA, Cutler GB, Loriauz DL. Petrosal sinus sampling with and without corticotrophin-releasing hormone for the differential diagnosis of Cushing's syndrome. *New England Journal of Medicine* 1991; 325: 897–905.

Orth DN. Cushing's syndrome *New England Journal of Medicine* 1995; 332: 791–803.

Chapter 20
Non-functioning pituitary tumours

Background

These pituitary tumours are unassociated with clinical syndromes of anterior pituitary hormone excess.

Epidemiology

- Non-functioning pituitary tumours (NFA) are the commonest pituitary macroadenoma. They represent 25% of all pituitary tumours.
- There is an equal sex distribution and the majority of cases present in patients aged >50 years.

Pathology

- Despite the fact that NFAs are unassociated with hormone production, they may immunostain for:
  - glycoprotein hormones (most commonly gonadotrophins) – LH, FSH, the α or β subunits or TSH
  - ACTH (silent corticotroph adenomas), or
  - be negative on immunostaining – either null cell tumours or oncocytomas (characteristically contain multiple mitochondria on electron microscopy).
- Tumour behaviour is variable, with some tumours behaving in a very indolent slow-growing manner and others invading the sphenoid and cavernous sinus.

Clinical features

Mass effects

* visual field defects (uni or bitemporal quadrantanopia or hemianopia)
* headache
* ophthalmoplegia (III, IV, and VI cranial nerves – rarely)
* optic atrophy (rarely, following long-term optic nerve compression)
* apoplexy (rarely).

Hypopituitarism

See page 113.

* At diagnosis, approximately 50% are gonadotrophin deficient.

Incidental finding

A NFA may be detected on the basis of imaging performed for other reasons.

Investigation

* *Pituitary imaging* MRI/CT demonstrates the tumour and/or invasion into the cavernous sinus or supraoptic recess.
* *Visual fields assessment* Abnormal in up to 2/3 of cases.
* *PRL* Essential to exclude a PRL secreting macroadenoma (see p. 139).
  – mild elevation (<3 000 mU/L) may occur secondary to stalk compression
  – borderline PRL 3000–6000 mU/L may warrant a trial of dopamine agonist treatment (see p. 224).
* *Pituitary function* Assessment for hypopituitarism (see p. 103).

Management

Surgery

+ The initial definitive management in virtually every case is surgical. This removes mass effects and may lead to some recovery of pituitary function in around 10%. The majority of patients can be operated on successfully via the trans-sphenoidal route.

+ Close follow-up is necessary after surgery as tumour regrowth can only be detected using pituitary imaging and visual field assessment, as there is no reliable consistent biochemical marker in the majority of cases.

Radiotherapy

+ The use of postoperative radiotherapy remains controversial. Some centres advocate its use for every patient following surgery; others reserve its use for those patients who have had particularly invasive or aggressive tumours removed or those with a significant amount of residual tumour remaining (e.g. in the cavernous sinus).

+ The regrowth rate at 10 years without radiotherapy approaches 45% and there are no good predictive factors for determining which tumours will regrow. However, administration of postoperative radiotherapy reduces this regrowth rate to less than 10%. As discussed in p. 220, however, there are sequelae to radiotherapy – with a significant long-term risk of hypopituitarism and a possible increased risk of visual deterioration and malignancy in the field of radiation.

Medical treatment

+ Unlike the case for GH and PRL-secreting tumours, medical therapy for NFAs is usually unhelpful, although there have been reports of the somatostatin agonist octreotide leading to tumour shrinkage and/or visual field improvement in some cases.

+ Hormone replacement therapy is required to treat any hypopituitarism (see p. 120).

Biochemical markers for NFAs?

* The majority of patients lack a hormone marker – despite approximately half immunostain positively for gonadotrophins and contain secretory granules at the EM level.

* A minority of patients have elevated circulating FSH/LH levels, see section on gonadotrophinomas (p. 182).

* The use of the response of α subunit or LH/FSH as a tumour marker has been suggested. Small series have shown that up to 70% of patients with functionless tumours show a 50% rise in serum gonadotrophin/subunit after 200 μg i/v TRH. As this response disappears after tumour resection it may be a useful tumour marker, although this is not widely practised.

Follow-up

* Patients who have not received postoperative irradiation require careful long-term follow-up with serial pituitary imaging and visual field assessment. The optimal protocol is still not known but an accepted practice is to image in the first 3 months following surgery and then re-image annually for 5 years and then biannually thereafter. Tumour recurrence has been reported at up to 15 years following surgery and therefore follow-up needs to be long-term.

* In patients who have received postoperative radiotherapy, follow-up with annual visual field assessment and imaging only if a deterioration is noted.

Prognosis

* Patients with NFAs have a good prognosis once the diagnosis and appropriate treatment including replacement of hormone deficiency is performed. The main concern is the risk of tumour regrowth with subsequent visual failure. As mentioned above, the administration of radiotherapy, although not without potential complications itself significantly reduces this risk. Unirradiated patients require very close follow-up in order to detect regrowth and perform repeat surgery or administer radiotherapy.

- Visual field defects at diagnosis may improve following surgery in the majority and improvement may continue for a year following tumour debulking.

Chapter 21
Gonadotrophinomas

Background

These are tumours that arise from the gonadotroph cells of the pituitary gland and produce FSH, LH, or the α subunit. They are often indistinguishable from other non-functioning pituitary adenomas as they are usually silent and unassociated with excess detectable secretion of LH and FSH, although studies demonstrate gonadotrophin/α subunit secretion *in vitro*. Occasionally however, these tumours do produce detectable excess hormone *in vivo*.

Clinical Features

Gonadotrophinomas present in the same manner as other non-functioning pituitary tumours with mass effects and hypopituitarism (see p. 177).

The rare FSH-secreting gonadotrophinomas may lead to macro-orchidism in men.

Investigation

The secretion of FSH and LH from these tumours is usually undetectable in the plasma. Occasionally elevated FSH and more rarely LH is measured. This finding is often ignored, particularly in post-menopausal women, although elevated gonadotrophins together with ACTH and/or TSH deficiency in the presence of a macroadenomas should raise the suspicion of a functioning gonadotrophinoma.

Management

These tumours are managed as non-functioning tumours. The potential advantage of FSH/LH secretion from a functioning gonadotrophinoma is that it provides a biochemical marker of presence of tumour for follow-up.

Chapter 22
Thyrotrophinomas

Epidemiology

These are rare tumours comprising approximately 1% of all pituitary tumours. The diagnosis may be delayed, because the significance of an unsuppressed TSH in the presence of elevated free thyroid hormone concentrations may be missed. Approximately 1/3 of cases in the literature have received treatment directed at the thyroid in the form of radioiodine treatment or surgery, before diagnosis.

Unlike primary hyperthyroidism, thyrotrophinomas are equally common in men and women.

Tumour biology and behaviour

- The majority are macroadenomas (90%) and secrete only TSH (72%), often with α-subunit in addition, but some co-secrete GH and/or PRL.
- The pathogenesis of thyrotoxicosis in the presence of normal TSH levels is poorly understood, but there are reports of secretion of TSH with increased bioactivity possibly due to changes in post-translational hormone glycosylation.
- The observation that prior thyroid ablation is associated with deleterious effects on the size of the tumour suggests some feedback control, and is similar to the aggressive tumours seen in Nelson's syndrome after bilateral adrenalectomy has been performed for Cushing's syndrome. Thyrotropin-secreting pituitary carcinoma has been very rarely reported.

Clinical features (see p. 46)

- Clinical features of *hyperthyroidism* are usually present, but often milder than expected given the level of thyroid hormones. In mixed tumours, hyperthyroidism may be overshadowed by features of *acromegaly*.
- *Mass effects* visual field defects and hypopituitarism

Investigation

- *TSH is inappropriately normal or elevated* The range of TSH that has been described is <1–568 mU/L, and 1/3 untreated patients had TSH in the normal range. There is no correlation between TSH and T_4.

- *Free thyroid hormones* elevated.

- *α-Subunit* Typically patients have an increased α-subunit : TSH molar ratio(>1).

- *Other anterior pituitary hormone levels* PRL and/or GH may be elevated in mixed tumours (an oral glucose tolerance test may be indicated to exclude acromegaly).

- *SHBG* elevated into the hyperthyroid range

- *TRH test* absent TSH response to stimulation with TRH (useful to differentiate TSH-secreting tumours from thyroid hormone resistance where the TSH response is normal or exaggerated).

- *Thyroid antibodies* In contrast to Graves' disease, the incidence of thyroid antibodies is similar to that in the general population.

- *Pituitary imaging* MRI scan will demonstrate a pituitary tumour (macroadenoma) in the majority of cases.

Causes of an elevated fT4 in the presence of an inappropriately unsuppressed TSH (see p. 46)

- TSH-secreting tumour
- thyroid hormone resistance
- amiodarone therapy
- inherited abnormalities of thyroid-binding proteins.

Management

Surgery

Surgery leads to cure in approximately 1/3 of patients as judged by apparent complete removal of tumour mass and normalization of thyroid hormone levels, with another 1/3 improved with normal thyroid hormone levels but incomplete removal of the adenoma.

Radiotherapy

Radiotherapy is useful following unsuccessful surgery, and leads to gradual (over years) reduction in TSH.

Medical treatment

Somatostatin analogues

• Medical treatment with the somatostatin agonists octreotide and lanreotide is successful in the majority of patients in suppressing TSH secretion and leading to tumour shrinkage. In one study, octreotide reduced TSH secretion in almost all patients treated, and normalized thyroid hormone levels in 73% of patients. There was partial tumour shrinkage in 40%.

• Drug therapy is useful in the preoperative preparation of these patients to ensure that they are fit for general anaesthetic and also while waiting for radiotherapy to be effective.

Anti-thyroid medication

• Treatment with antithyroid drugs has been associated with increased TSH in approximately 60% of patients reported. It should be avoided if possible and the more appropriate somatostatin agonist therapy utilized.

Further reading

Beck-Peccoz P, Brucker-Davis F Persani L, Smallridge RC, Weintraub BD. Thyrotropin-secreting pituitary tumours. *Endocrine Reviews* 1996;17: 610–638.

Chanson P, Weintraub BD, Harris AG. Octreotide therapy for thyroid stimulating hormone-secreting pituitary adenomas. *Annals of Internal Medicine* 1993;119: 236–240.

Chapter 23
Pituitary incidentalomas

Definition

The term incidentaloma refers to an incidentally detected lesion that is unassociated with hormonal hyper or hyposecretion and has a benign natural history.

The increasingly frequent detection of these lesions with technological improvements and more widespread use of sophisticated imaging has led to a management challenge – which, if any lesions need investigation and/or treatment, and what is the optimal follow-up strategy (if required at all)?

Epidemiology

* Autopsy studies have shown that 10–20% of pituitary glands unsuspected of having pituitary disease harbour pituitary adenomas. Approximately half the tumours stain for PRL and the remainder are negative on immunostaining.
* Imaging studies using MRI demonstrate pituitary microadenomas in approximately 10% of normal volunteers.
* Incidentally detected macroadenomas have been reported when imaging has been performed for other reasons. However, these are not true incidentalomas as they are often associated with visual field defects, and/or hypopituitarism.

Natural history

Incidentally detected microadenomas are very unlikely to increase in size (<10%) whereas larger incidentally detected meso- and macroadenomas are more likely to enlarge (30%).

Clinical features

By definition, a patient with an incidentaloma should be asymptomatic. Any patient who has an incidentally detected tumour should have visual field assessment and a clinical review to ensure that this is not the initial presentation of Cushing's syndrome or acromegaly.

Investigation

- Aims:
  - exclude any hormone hypersecretion from the tumour
  - detect hypopituitarism.
- Investigation of hypersecretion of hormones should include measurement of PRL, IGF-1, and an oral glucose tolerance test if acromegaly is suspected, 24 h urinary free cortisol and overnight dexamethasone suppression test and thyroid function tests (unsuppressed TSH in the presence of elevated T_4).
- Others suggest that this approach is unnecessary, but with limited data most endocrinologists would perform investigations as above.

Management

- All extra-sellar macroadenomas (incidentally detected but by definition not true incidentalomas) require definitive treatment.
- Tumours with excess hormone secretion require definitive treatment.
- Mass <1 cm repeat MRI at 1, 2, and 5 years.
- Mass >1 cm diameter – repeat MRI at 6 months, 1, 2, and 5 years.

Further reading

Turner HE, Moore NR, Byrne JV, Wass JAH. Pituitary, adrenal and thyroid incidentalomas. *Endocrine-related Cancer* 1998; 5: 131–150.

Chapter 24
Pituitary carcinoma

Definition

Pituitary carcinoma is defined as a primary adenohypophyseal neoplasm with craniospinal and/or distant systemic metastases.

Epidemiology

These are extremely rare tumours, and only approximately 60 cases have been reported in the world literature.

Pathology and pathogenesis

- The initial tumours and subsequent carcinomas show higher proliferation indices than the majority of pituitary adenomas. They are also likely to demonstrate p53 positivity and have an increased mitotic index.
- The aetiology of these tumours is unknown, but the adenoma–carcinoma sequence is followed in ACTH-secreting tumours:- pituitary adenoma causing Cushing's disease, followed by locally invasive adenoma (Nelson's syndrome) leading to pituitary carcinoma.

Features

Virtually all pituitary carcinomas initially present as invasive pituitary macroadenomas. After a variable interval of time (mean 6.5 years) the majority present with local recurrence. There is a tendency to systemic (liver, lymph nodes, lungs, and bones) rather than craniospinal metastases but metastases do not usually predominate in the clinical picture.

Table 24.1 Types of pituitary carcinoma

Type	Proportion of reported cases
PRL	30%
ACTH	28%
GH	2%
Non-functioning	30%

NB Many 'non-functioning' carcinomas were reported prior to routine measurement of PRL or routine immunostaining, and therefore the true incidence of PRL-producing carcinomas may be higher.

Treatment

Radiotherapy or medical treatment provide palliation only.

Further reading

Pernicone PJ, Scheithauer BW, Sebo TJ, Kovacs KT, Horvath E, Young WF, LLoyd RV, Davis DH, Guthrie BL, Schoene WC. Pituitary carcinoma. *Cancer* 1997;79: 804–812.

Chapter 25

Craniopharyngiomas and perisellar cysts

Incidence

1–2/million/year

Epidemiology

Any age, only 50% present in childhood (<16 years).

Pathology

Tumour arising from squamous epithelial remnants of Rathke's pouch. Histology may be either adamantinous epithelial, with cyst formation and calcification, or squamous papillary (generally associated with a better prognosis). Cyst formation and calcification is common. Benign tumour, although infiltrates surrounding structures. hCG is present in cyst fluid.

Rathke's cleft cysts

Pathology

Derived from the remnants of Rathke's pouch, lined by epithelial cells and filled with fluid. (Ciliated cuboidal/columnar epithelium, compared with squamous for craniopharyngiomas.)

Features

Usually asymptomatic, although may present with headache and amenorrhoea, and rarely hypopituitarism and hydrocephalus.

Investigation

CT/MRI – variable enhancement.

Management

* Decompression if symptomatic.
* Recurrence is rare.

Other perisellar cysts

* Arachnoid
* Epidermoid
* Dermoid

Features

- raised intracranial pressure
- visual disturbance
- hypothalamopituitary disturbance
  – growth failure in children
  – precocious puberty and tall stature are less common
  – anterior and posterior pituitary failure, including DI.

Investigation

- MRI/CT (CT may be helpful to evaluate boney erosion)
- visual field assessment
- anterior and posterior pituitary assessment (p. 113).

Management

Surgery is the primary treatment for the majority, usually trans-cranial, occasionally trans-sphenoidal.

The extent of surgery is variable – high risk of recurrence leads some to recommend radical surgery, but high postoperative morbidity, e.g. hypothalamic syndrome, has led many neurosurgeons to recommend subtotal removal and postoperative radiotherapy.

Chapter 26
Parasellar tumours

Meningiomas

- Suprasellar meningiomas arise from the tuberculum sellae or the chiasmal sulcus.
- Usually present with a chiasmal syndrome where loss of visual acuity occurs in one eye followed by reduced acuity in the other eye.
- Differentiation from a primary pituitary tumour can be difficult where there is downward extension into the sella.
- MRI is the imaging of choice. T1 weighted images demonstrate meningiomas as isodense with grey matter and hypointense with respect to pituitary tissue, with marked enhancement after gadolinium.
- Cerebral angiography also demonstrates a tumour blush.
- Management is surgical and may also be complicated by haemorrhage as these are often very vascular tumours. They are relatively radioresistant but inoperable or partially removed tumours may respond. As they are slow-growing, a conservative approach with regular imaging may be appropriate.
- Associations include type 2 neurofibromatosis.

Clivus chordomas

- Rare. Arise from embryonic rest cells of the notochord.
- May present with cranial nerve palsies (III, VI, IX, X) or pyramidal tract dysfunction.
- Anterior and posterior pituitary hypofunction is reported.
- Often invasive and relentlessly progressive.
- Treatment is surgical followed by radiotherapy in some cases, although they are relatively radioresistant. Data on radiosurgery are not yet available, but this may be considered.

Hamartomas

- Non-neoplastic overgrowth of neurones and glial cells.
- Rare. May present with seizures – typically gelastic (laughing).
- May release GnRH leading to precocious puberty or very rarely GHRH leading to disorders of growth or acromegaly.
- Appear as homogeneous isointense with grey matter, pedunculated or sessile non-enhancing tumours on T1 weighted MRI scans.

Management

Tumours do not enlarge, and therefore treatment is of endocrine consequences – most commonly precocious puberty.

Ependymomas

- Intracranial ependymomas typically affect children and adolescents.
- Pituitary insufficiency may follow craniospinal irradiation.
- Occasionally third ventricle tumours may interfere with hypothalamic function.

Secondary neoplasm

- Patients particularly with breast or bronchial carcinoma may present with secondaries usually in the hypothalamus or in the pituitary itself.
  DI is common.

Chapter 27
Parasellar inflammatory conditions

Neurosarcoidosis

Pituitary and hypothalamus may be affected by meningeal disease. Most patients with hypothalamic sarcoidosis also have involvement outside the CNS.

Features

Hypopituitarism and DI, in addition to hypothalamic syndrome of absent thirst, somnolence, and hyperphagia.

Investigations

- Serum and CSF ACE may be raised.
- CSF examination may reveal a pleocytosis, oligoclonal bands, and low glucose.
- MRI may demonstrate additional enhancement, e.g. meningeal.
- Gallium scan may reveal increased uptake in lacrimal and salivary glands.

Management

- High doses of glucocorticoids (60–80 mg prednisolone) for initial treatment. Subsequent treatment with 40 mg/day is often required for several months. Pulsed methylprednisolone may also be useful. Steroid sparing agents such as azathioprine may be helpful.
- Management of hormonal deficiency can be very difficult particularly in the context of absent thirst and poor memory.

Langerhans' cell histiocytosis

• Over 50% of cases occur in children.
• Most frequent endocrine abnormalities are DI and growth retardation due to hypothalamic infiltration by Langerhans' cells or involvement of the meninges adjacent to the pituitary. Rarely hyperprolactinaemia and panhypopituitarism develop. In adults, DI may precede the bone and soft tissue abnormalities making diagnosis difficult.

Management

The role of radiotherapy is controversial, with some workers reporting improvement, and others questioning the efficacy. If radiotherapy is used, rapid institution of treatment appears to be important (within 10 days of diagnosis). High dose glucocorticoids can lead to transient improvement, but chemotherapy does not alter the course of DI although it may lead to temporary regression of lesions.

Tuberculosis

TB may present as a tuberculoma which may compromise hypothalamic or pituitary function. DI is common. Most patients have signs of TB elsewhere, but not invariably so. Trans-sphenoidal biopsy is therefore sometimes required. An alternative strategy is antituberculous treatment with empirical glucocorticoid treatment.

Further reading

Freda PU, Post KD. Differential diagnosis of sellar masses. *Endocrinology and Metabolism Clinics of North America* 1999; 28: 81.

Chapter 28
Lymphocytic hypophysitis

Background

This is a rare inflammatory condition of the pituitary.

Epidemiology

Lymphocytic hypophysitis occurs more commonly in women, and usually presents during late pregnancy or the first year thereafter.

Pathogenesis

Ill-understood – probably autoimmune. Approximately 25% of cases of lymphocytic hypophysitis have been associated with other auto-immune conditions – Hashimoto's thyroiditis in the majority, but also pernicious anaemia

Pathology

- Somatotroph and gonadotroph function are more likely to be preserved than corticotroph or thyrotroph function, unlike the findings in hypopituitarism due to a pituitary tumour. The posterior pituitary is characteristically spared so that DI is not part of the picture, but there are occasional reports of coexistent or isolated DI, presumably because of different antigens.
- Lymphocytic hypophysitis has occasionally involved the cavernous sinus and extra-ocular muscles.
- Light microscopy typically reveals a lymphoplasmacytic infiltrate, occasionally forming lymphoid follicles, with variable destruction of parenchyma and fibrosis.

Clinical features

- Mass effects leading to headache and visual field defects.
- Often a temporal association with pregnancy.
- Hypopituitarism (ACTH and TSH deficiency, less commonly gonadotrophin and GH deficiency).
- Posterior pituitary involvement and cavernous sinus involvement occur less commonly.

Investigations

- Investigation of hypopituitarism is essential, and may not be thought of because gonadotrophin secretion often remains intact, leaving the potentially life-threatening ACTH deficiency unsuspected.
- MRI shows an enhancing mass, with variably loss of hyperintense bright spot of neurohypophysis, thickening of pituitary stalk, enlargement of the neurohypophysis. Suprasellar extension often appears tongue-like along the pituitary stalk. There may be central necrosis but no calcification.
- Biopsy of the lesion is often required, but may be avoided in the presence of typical features.
- The presence of antipituitary antibodies has been investigated by some groups and shown to be variably present. This is, however, a research tool and an unreliable marker.

Table 28.1 Classification of hypophysitis

Acute	Bacterial infections
Chronic	Lymphocytic hypophysitis
	Xanthomatous (characterized by lipid-laden macrophages)
Granulomatous	Tuberculosis
	Sarcoidosis
	Syphilis
	Giant cell (? variant of lymphocytic hypophysitis)

Treatment

- Treatment of hypopituitarism.
- Most often, no specific treatment is necessary. There is anecdotal evidence only of the effectiveness of immunosupressive doses of glucocorticoids – for example prednisolone 60 mg /day for 3 months and progressive reduction for 6 months. This has been reported to be associated with reduction in the mass and gradual recovery of pituitary function. However, relapse after discontinuing therapy is also reported.
- Spontaneous recovery may also occur.
- Surgery has also been used to improve visual field abnormalities

Natural history

Variable – some progress rapidly to life-threatening hypopituitarism, while others spontaneously regress.

Relationship to other conditions

Lymphocytic hypophysitis remains an ill-understood condition but has been suggested to be the underlying cause of other conditions such as isolated ACTH deficiency and the empty sella syndrome.

Further reading

Thodou *et al. Journal of Clinical Endocrinology and Metabolism* 1995; 80: 2302–2311.

Thodoy E, Asa SL, Kontogeorgos G, Kovacs K, Harvath E, Ezzat S Clinical case seminar: lymphocytic hypophysitis: clinicopathological findings.

Chapter 29
Surgical treatment of
pituitary tumours

Trans-sphenoidal surgery

This is now the favoured technique for pituitary surgery, and is first line for virtually every case. It is preferred to the previously used technique of craniotomy because there is minimal associated morbidity as a result of the fact that the cranial fossa is not opened and there are therefore no immediate sequelae due to direct cerebral damage (particularly frontal lobe) and no long-term risk of epilepsy. There is reduced duration of hospital stay and improved cure rates as there is better visualization of small tumours. Unfortunately the technique may be inadequate to deal with very large tumours with extensive suprasellar extension. In these situations craniotomy is required if adequate debulking is not possible following the trans-sphenoidal approach.

Preparation for trans-sphenoidal surgery

Pretreatment before surgery

- Pretreatment with *metyrapone* or *ketoconazole* to improve the condition of patients with Cushing's syndrome is often given for at least 6 weeks. This allows some improvement in healing and also improves the general state of the patient.

- Patients with macroprolactinomas will in the majority of cases have received treatment with dopamine agonists in any case, and surgery is usually indicated for resistance of intolerance. There is a risk of tumour fibrosis, with long-term (>6/12) dopamine agonist therapy.

Immediately preoperative

- Immediate preoperative treatment requires appropriate anterior pituitary hormone replacement. In particular, a decision as to whether perioperative glucocorticoid treatment is required. The majority of microprolactinomas will not require perioperative hydrocortisone, but patients with Cushing's syndrome will require peri-and postoperative glucocorticoid treatment (see p. 784). Patients with macroadenomas and an intact preoperative pituitary–adrenal axis do not usually require perioperative steroids, but those who are deficient or whose reserve has not been tested need to be given perioperative glucocorticoids. TSH deficiency should be corrected with thyroxine.

- Prophylactic antibiotics are started in some centres the night before surgery to reduce the chances of meningitis.

Complications

See table on p. 214.

* Patients should be counselled about the possible complications of trans-sphenoidal surgery prior to consent. The commonest complications are DI which may be transient or permanent (5% and 0.1% respectively; often higher in Cushing's disease and prolactinoma) and the development of new anterior pituitary hormonal deficiencies (uncommon with microadenomas, approximately 10% of TSA for macroadenomas).

* The risk of meningitis can be reduced by preoperative and perioperative prophylactic antibiotic administration. In Oxford our practice is to give 5 days of oral antibiotics (*amoxycillin* and *flucloxacillin*, or *erythromycin* if penicillin allergic) starting the night before surgery. Other complications include CSF leak, visual deterioration, haemorrhage (rare), and transient hyponatraemia usually 7 days postoperatively.

Indications

* non-functioning pituitary adenoma
* GH-secreting adenoma
* ACTH secreting tumour
* Nelson's syndrome
* prolactinoma (if patient dopamine agonist resistant or intolerant)
* recurrent pituitary tumour

Less common

* gonadotrophin-secreting tumours
* TSH-secreting adenoma
* craniopharyngioma
* pituitary biopsy to define diagnosis e.g. hypophysitis, pituitary metastases
* chordoma
* Rathke's cleft cyst
* arachnoid cyst

Table 29.1 Complications of trans-spenoidal surgery

Complications of any surgical procedure	Anaesthetic related
	Venous thrombosis and pulmonary embolism
Immediate	Haemorrhage
	Hypothalamic damage
	Meningitis
Permanent	Visual deterioration or loss
	Cranial nerve damage (e.g. oculomotor nerve palsies)
	Hypopituitarism
	DI
	SIADH
Transient	DI
	CSF rhinorrhoea
	Visual deterioration
	Cerebral salt wasting

Cerebral salt wasting

A rare but important complication of trans-sphenoidal surgery, that is more commonly seen after subarachnoid haemorrhage is cerebral salt wasting syndrome (CSW). This typically occurs at day 5–10 postoperatively and is associated with often massive urinary salt loss, and hypovolaemia. It needs to be differentiated from SIADH which may also occur at this stage (often using central venous pressure measurement to demonstrate hypovolaemia in CSW compared with euvolaemia in SIADH). The management of CSW involves administration of saline, whereas fluid restriction is indicated for SIADH.

Trans-frontal craniotomy

Indications

- Pituitary tumours with major suprasellar and lateral invasion where trans-sphenoidal surgery is unlikely to remove a significant proportion of the tumour.
- Craniopharyngiomas.
- Parasellar tumours, e.g. meningioma.

Complications

- In addition to the complications of trans-sphenoidal surgery, brain retraction leads to cerebral oedema or haemorrhage.
- Manipulation of the optic chiasm may lead to visual deterioration.
- Vascular damage.
- Damage to the olfactory nerve.

Perioperative management

Similar to that for patients undergoing trans-sphenoidal surgery.

Postoperative management

- Recovery is typically slower than after trans-sphenoidal surgery.
- Prophylactic anticonvulsants are administered for up to 1 year.
- The DVLC must be advised of surgery, and driving is allowed following adequate visual recovery, but drivers of group 2 vehicles (HGV) cannot drive for 6 months.

Further reading

Laws ER, Thapar K. Pituitary surgery. *Endocrinology and Metabolism Clinics of North America* 1999; 28: 119.

Chapter 30
Pituitary radiotherapy

Indications

See table on facing page.

- Pituitary radiotherapy is an effective treatment used to reduce the liklihood of tumour regrowth, to further shrink a tumour, and to treat persistent hormone hypersecretion following surgical resection.

- Occasionally it is used as a primary therapeutic option, but its usual role is following non-curative surgery or following macroprolactinoma shrinkage with dopamine agonists.

- Pituitary radiotherapy is usually only administrable once in a lifetime.

Technique

- Conventional external beam three-field radiotherapy is able to deliver a beam of ionizing irradiation accurately to the pituitary fossa.

- Accurate targeting requires head fixation in a moulded plastic shell to keep the head immobilized. The fields of irradiation are based on simulation using MRI or CT scanning and the volume is usually the tumour margins plus 0.5 cm in all planes. The preoperative tumour volume is used for planning, whereas the post-drug (dopamine agonist) shrinkage films are used for prolactinomas. There are three portals, two temporal and one anterior.

- The standard dose is 4500 cGy in 25 fractions over 35 days, but 5000 cGy may be used for relatively 'radioresistant' tumours such as craniopharyngiomas.

Efficacy

Radiotherapy is effective in reducing the chances of pituitary tumour regrowth. For example, in a large series of 400 patients who received pituitary radiotherapy over a period of 20 years, the progression-free survival rate was 97% at 10 years and 92% at 20 years. Comparison of functionless tumour recurrence following surgery and radiotherapy compared with surgery alone, shows that radiotherapy is effective in reducing the likelihood of regrowth (Figure 30.1).

Table 30.1 Indications for pituitary radiotherapy

Tumour	Aim of treatment
Non-functioning pituitary adenoma	To shrink residual mass or reduce liklihood of regrowth
GH/PRL/ACTH secreting tumour	To reduce persistent hormonal hypersecretion and shrink residual mass
Craniopharyngioma	To reduce likelihood of regrowth
Recurrent tumour	

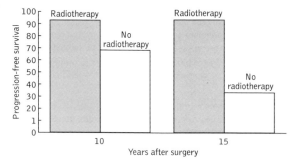

Fig. 30.1 Recurrence rates following radiotherapy. (Modified from Gittoes NJL, Bates AS, Tse W *et al.* Radiotherapy for non-functioning pituitary tumours. *Clinical Endocrinology* 1998; 48: 331–7).

Complications

Short term

* nausea
* headache
* temporary hair loss at radiotherapy portals of entry.

Hypopituitarism

* Anterior pituitary hormone deficiency occurs due to the effect of irradiation on the hypothalamus leading to reduced hypothalamic releasing hormone secretion. The total dose of irradiation determines the speed, incidence and extent of hypopituitarism. In addition the presence of pre-existing hormonal deficiency increases the chances of post-radiotherapy hypopituitarism (Table 30.2).

* The onset of hypopituitarism is gradual, and the order of development of deficiency is as for any other cause of developing hypopituitarism – namely GH first followed by gonadotrophin and ACTH followed finally by TSH. Posterior pituitary deficiencies are very rare, but secondary temporary mild hyperprolactinaemia may be seen after about 2 years which gradually returns to normal.

Visual impairment

* The optic chiasm is particularly radioresistant, but may undergo damage thought to be due to vascular damage to the blood supply. Visual deterioration typically occurs within 3 years of irradiation, and is progressive.

* The literature suggest that the risk is greatest with high total and daily doses. A standard total dose of 4500 cGy and daily dose of 180 cGy appears to pose very little, if any, risk to the chiasm.

* Our practice is to avoid administration of radiotherapy where possible when the chiasm is under pressure from residual tumour.

Radiation oncogenesis

* There is controversy as to whether pituitary irradiation leads to the development of second tumours. There have been reports of sarcomas, gliomas and meningiomas developing in the field of irradiation after 10–20 years. However, there are also reports of gliomas and meningioma occurring in unirradiated patients with pituitary adenomas. A retrospective review of a large series of patients given pituitary irradiation suggested a risk of second tumour of 1.9% by

20 years after irradiation when compared to the normal population (but not patients with pituitary tumours).

- More subtle changes in neurocognition have been suggested.

Table 30.2 Development of new hypopituitarism at 10 years following pituitary radiotherapy

	No previous surgery	Surgery
Gonadotrophin deficiency	47%	70%
ACTH deficiency	30%	54%
Thyrotrophin deficiency	16%	38%

Focal forms of radiotherapy

Stereotactic radiosurgery uses focused radiation to deliver a precise dose of radiation:

- Gamma knife 'radiosurgery' – ionizing radiation from a cobalt 60 source delivered by convergent collimated beams

- Linear accelerator focal radiotherapy – photons focused on a stationary point from a moving gantry

- Potential advantages are that a single high dose of irradiation is given which can be sharply focused on the tumour with minimal surrounding tissue damage.

- Long-term data are required to demonstrate endocrine efficacy, but it may have a particular role in recurrent or persistent tumours which are well-demarcated and surgically inaccessible e.g. in the cavernous sinus.

- Potential limitations include proximity to the optic chiasm.

Further reading

Brada M, Ford D, Ashley S *et al.* Risk of second brain tumour after conservative surgery and radiotherapy for pituitary adenoma. *BMJ* 1992; 304: 1343–1346.

Jackson IMD, Noren G. Role of gamma knife therapy in the management of pituitary tumours. *Endocrinology and Metabolism Clinics of North America* 1999; 28: 133.

Jones A. Radiation oncogenesis in relation to treatment of pituitary tumours. *Clinical Endocrinology* 1991; 35: 379

Plowman PN. Pituitary adenoma radiotherapy. *Clinical Endocrinology* 1999; 51: 265–271.

Chapter 31
Drug treatment of
pituitary tumours

Dopamine agonists

Types

* *Bromocriptine* The first ergot alkaloid to be used, short acting, taken daily. Usually administered orally, although vaginal and i/m formulations can be used and may reduce gastrointestinal intolerance.

* *Quinagolide* Non-ergot, longer acting, taken daily.

* *Cabergoline* Ergot derivative. Long acting – taken once or twice a week.

* *Less commonly used* pergolide and lisuride.

Mechanism of action

Activation of D2 receptors.

Side-effects

Commonly at initiation of treatment

* nausea
* postural hypotension

Less common

* Headache, fatigue, nasal stuffiness, constipation, abdominal cramps, and a Raynaud like phenomenon in hands.

* Very rarely patients have developed hallucinations and psychosis (usually at higher doses).

* Side-effects may be minimized by slow initiation of therapy (e.g. 1.25 mg bromocriptine or 0.25 mg cabergoline), taking medication before going to bed, and taking the tablets with food.

Uses

Hyperprolactinaemia (see p. 136)

* D2 receptor stimulation leads to inhibition of PRL secretion and reduction in cell size leading to tumour shrinkage. The PRL often falls before significant tumour shrinkage is seen.

* Problems may arise when patients are either intolerant of the medication or resistant. Cabergoline appears to be better tolerated than bromocriptine and it is often worth trying an alternative in the case of intolerance, although true intolerance is probably a class effect. Dopamine agonist resistance (10–25% patients) may be due to dif-

ferences in receptor subtype (e.g. loss of D2 receptors) or possibly altered intracellular signalling.

GH-secreting tumours

- Although administration of L-dopa to normal individuals leads to acute increase in GH due to hypothalamic dopamine and noradrenaline synthesis and inhibition of somatostatin secretion, over half of patients with GH-secreting tumours given dopamine agonists have a fall in GH. Dopamine acts directly on somatotroph tumours to inhibit GH release.

- Patients with acromegaly often need larger doses of dopamine agonist than patients with prolactinomas. Tumour shrinkage is most likely if there is concomitant secretion of PRL from the tumour. Dopamine agonists are currently usually reserved for second line drug therapy in patients who are somatostatin agonist resistant or as a co-prescription with somatostatin agonists in patients with mixed GH-and PRL-secreting tumours.

Pregnancy

Bromocriptine is licensed for use in pregnancy, but cabergoline is not licensed in the UK, although it has not thus far been associated with any increased teratogeneicity.

Somatostatin analogues

Mechanism of action

- Since the half-life of somatostatin is very short, a longer acting analogue was synthesized – octreotide. This has a half-life of 110 min in the circulation, inhibits GH secretion 45 times more actively than native somatostatin, with none of the rebound hypersecretion that occurs with somatostatin.
- The somatostatin analogues act predominantly on the somatostatin receptors 2 and 5. Unlike dopamine agonists, somatostatin analogues do not lead to dramatic tumour shrinkage, but some shrinkage is still seen in the majority of tumours.

Types

- S/c octreotide (50–200 μg)   administered 3× daily
- Lanreotide SR (30 mg i/m)   administered every 7–14 days
- Octreotide LAR (10–30 mg i/m)   administered every 4–6 weeks.
- Lanreotide autogel (60–120 mg i/m)   administered every 4 weeks.

Side-effects

- Gallstones At least 20–30% of patients develop gallstones or sludge on octreotide (thought by most to antedate stone formation), but only 1%/year develop symptoms. The incidence is unknown on octreotide LAR or Lanreotide.
- Gastrointestinal due to inhibition of motor activity and secretion leading to nausea, abdominal cramps, and mild steatorrhoea. These usually settle with time.
- Injection site pain Obviated by allowing vial to warm to room temperature before injecting.

Uses (see relevant section)

- acromegaly
- carcinoid tumours
- pancreatic neuroendocrine tumours
- TSH-secreting pituitary tumours
- non-functioning pituitary tumours.

Chapter 32
Posterior pituitary

Physiology and pathology

The posterior lobe of the pituitary gland arises from the forebrain, and comprises up to 25% of the normal adult pituitary gland. It produces arginine vasopressin and oxytocin. Both hormones are synthesized in the hypothalamic neurons of the supra-optic and paraventricular nuclei and migrate as neurosecretory granules to the posterior pituitary before release into the circulation. The hormones are unbound in the circulation and their half-life is short.

Oxytocin

- Oxytocin has no known role in men. It may aid contraction of the seminal vesicles.
- In women, oxytocin contracts the pregnant uterus and also causes breast duct smooth muscle contraction leading to breast-milk ejection during breast-feeding. Oxytocin is released in response to suckling and also to cervical dilatation during parturition. However, oxytocin deficiency has no known adverse effect on parturition or breast-feeding.
- There are several as yet ill-understood features of oxytocin physiology. For example, osmotic stimulation may also lead to oxytocin secretion. Oxytocin may play a role in the ovary and testis, as ovarian luteal cells and testicular cells have both been shown to synthesize it, although its subsequent role is not known.

Vasopressin and neurophysin

- Arginine vasopressin is the major determinant of renal water excretion and therefore fluid balance. Its main action is to reduce free water clearance.

- Vasopressin is a nonapeptide, and derives from a large precursor – with a signal peptide, and a neurophysin. The vasopressin gene is located on chromosome 20, and is closely linked to the oxytocin gene. Vasopressin travels to the posterior pituitary at about 2 mm/h, and undergoes cleavage as it travels. Neurophysin is released with vasopressin but has no further role after acting as a carrier protein in the neurons.

- Release of vasopressin occurs in response to changes in osmolality detected by osmoreceptors in the hypothalamus. Large changes in blood volume (5–10%) also influence vasopressin secretion. Many substances modulate vasopressin secretion including the catecholamines and opioids.

- The main site of action of vasopressin is in the collecting duct and the thick ascending loop of Henle where it increases water permeability so that solute free water may pass along an osmotic gradient to the interstitial medulla. Vasopressin in higher concentrations has a pressor effect. It also acts as an ACTH secretagogue synergistically with CRH.

Chapter 33
Diabetes insipidus

Definition

DI is defined as the passage of large volumes (>3 litre/24 h) of dilute urine (osmolality <300 mOsmol/kg).

Classification

Cranial
Due to deficiency of circulating arginine vasopressin (anti-diuretic hormone)

Nephrogenic
Due to renal resistance to vasopressin.

Primary polydipsia
• Polyuria due to excessive drinking.
• In addition to suppressed levels of vasopressin due to low plasma osmolality, there may be impaired renal effectiveness because of wash out of solute and therefore reduced urine-concentrating ability.

Features

• *Adults* polyuria, nocturia, and thirst
• *Children* polyuria, enuresis, and failure to thrive
• NB Clinical syndrome of cranial DI may be masked by cortisol deficiency as this results in failure to excrete a water load.
• Syndrome may worsen in pregnancy due to placental breakdown (vasopressinase) of circulating vasopressin.

Causes of DI

Cranial

10% vasopressin cells should be sufficient to keep the urine volume <4l/day.

Familial

* autosomal dominant (vasopressin gene)
* DIDMOAD syndrome (DI, diabetes mellitus, optic atrophy, deafness).

Acquired

* trauma (head injury, neurosurgery)
* tumours (craniopharyngiomas, pituitary infiltration by metastases)
* inflammatory conditions (sarcoidosis, tuberculosis, Langerhans cell histiocytosis, lymphocytic hypophysitis)
* infections (meningitis, encephalitis)
* vascular (Sheehan's syndrome, sickle cell disease)
* idiopathic.

Nephrogenic

Familial

* X-linked recessive (vasopressin receptor gene)
* autosomal recessive (aquaporin-2 gene).

Acquired

* drugs (lithium, demeclocycline)
* metabolic (hypercalcaemia, hypokalaemia, hyperglycaemia)
* chronic renal disease
* post-obstructive uropathy.

Primary polydipsia

* psychological.

Investigation

Diagnosis of type of DI

- Confirm large urine output (> 3000 mL/day).
- Exclude diabetes mellitus and renal failure (osmotic diuresis).
- Check electrolytes. Hypokalaemia and hypercalcaemia (nephrogenic DI).
- Fluid deprivation test (see p. 235) and assessment of response to vasopressin.
- Occasionally further investigations are required, particularly when only partial forms of the condition are present;
- Measurement of plasma vasopressin, osmolality, and thirst threshold:
  - in response to infusion of 0.05 mL/kg per min 5% hypertonic saline for 2 h for cranial DI (no increased vasopressin)
  - in response to fluid deprivation for nephrogenic DI (vasopressin levels rise with no increased urine osmolality).
- An alternative is a therapeutic trial of desmopressin with monitoring of sodium and osmolality.

Investigation of the cause

- MRI head
  - looking for tumours – hypothalamic, pineal, or infiltration
  - often demonstrates loss of bright spot of posterior pituitary gland.
- Serum ACE (sarcoidosis) and tumour markers, e.g. βHCG (pineal germinoma).

Fluid deprivation test

1 Patient is allowed fluids overnight. If psychogenic polydipsia suspected, consider overnight fluid deprivation to avoid morning overhydration).

2 Patient is then deprived of fluids for 8 h or until 5% loss of body weight if earlier. Weigh patient hourly.

3 Plasma osmolality is measured 4 hourly and urine volume and osmolality every 2 h.

4 The patient is then given 2 μg i/m desmopressin with urine volume, and urine and serum osmolality measured over the next 4 h.

Results

If serum osmolality >305 mOsm/kg – patient has DI and test is stopped.

Urine osmolality (Osm/kg)

Diagnosis	After fluid deprivation	After desmopressin
Cranial DI	<300	>800
Nephrogenic DI	<300	<300
Primary polydipsia	>800	>800
Partial DI or polydipsia	300–800	<800

Treatment

Maintenance of adequate fluid input
In patients with partial DI, and an intact thirst mechanism, then drug therapy may not be necessary if the polyuria is mild (<4l/24 h).

Drug therapy

Desmopressin
• Vasopressin analogue, acting predominantly on the V2 receptors in the kidney, with little action on the V1 receptors of blood vessels. It thus has reduced pressor activity and increased antidiuretic efficacy, in addition to a longer half-life than the native hormone.
• Drug may be administered in divided doses, orally (100–1000 μg/day), intranasally (10–40 μg/day) or parenterally (s/c, i/v, im) (0.1–2 μg/day). There is wide variation in the dose required by an individual patient.
• Monitoring of serum sodium and osmolality is essential as hyponatraemia or hypo-osmolality may develop.

Lysine vasopressin
• The antidiuretic hormone of the pig family.
• Not used very often as its effects are short lived (1–3 h) and it may retain pressor activity. Intranasal administration. Dose 5–20 U/day.

Chlorpropamide (100–500 mg/day) and carbamazepine enhance the action of vasopressin on the collecting duct.

Nephrogenic DI
• Correction of underlying cause (metabolic or drugs).
• High doses of desmopressin (e.g. up to 5 μg i/m) can be effective.
• Maintenance of adequate fluid input.
• Thiazide diuretics and prostaglandin synthase inhibitors (decrease the action of prostaglandins which locally inhibit the action of vasopressin in the kidney), e.g. indomethacin, can be helpful.

Polydipsic polyuria
Management is difficult. Treatment of any underlying psychiatric disorder is important.

Chapter 34
Hyponatraemia

Causes

Excess water (dilutional)

- excess water intake
- increased water reabsorption (cirrhosis, congestive cardiac failure, nephrotic syndrome)
- reduced renal excretion of a water load (SIADH, glucocorticoid deficiency)

Salt deficiency

- Renal loss (salt wasting nephropathy – tubulointerstitial nephritis, polycystic kidney disease, analgesic nephropathy, recovery phase of acute tubular necrosis, relief of bilateral ureteric obstruction).
- Non-renal loss (skin, gastrointestinal tract [bowel sequestration, high fistulae]).
- Renal sodium conservation of sodium is efficient and therefore low salt intake alone never causes sodium deficiency.

Pseudohyponatraemia

- Lipids, proteins (e.g. paraproteinaemia)
- Sodium only in aqueous phase of plasma, therefore, depending on assay, total sodium concentration may be spuriously low if concentrations of lipid or protein are high.

Solute

- Glucose, mannitol, ethanol.
- Addition of solute confined to the ECF causes water to shift from the ICF lowering ECF sodium concentration.

Sick cell syndrome

- Symptomless hyponatraemia at 120–130 mmol/L
- True clinically apparent hyponatraemia is associated with either excess water or salt deficiency. The other causes can usually be easily excluded.

Table 34.1 Hyponatraemia

Hypovolaemic		Euvolaemic		Hypervolaemic	
NaU >20 mmol/L	NaU <20 mmol/L	NaU <20 mmol/L	NaU >20 mmol/L, Serum osmolality <270 mOsm/kg, Urine osmolality >100 mOsm/kg	NaU <20 mmol/L	NaU >20 mmol/L, Serum osmolality <270 mOsm/kg, Urine osmolality >100 mOsm/kg
Renal sodium loss	Non-renal sodium loss	Depletional ECF loss with inappropriate fluid replacement	Distal dilution	Excess water	
?Salt losing nephropathy	?GIT loss		SIADH	Cirrhosis	SIADH
?Mineralocorticoid deficiency	?Skin loss		GC deficiency	Nephrotic syndrome	
				CCF	

GC = glucocorticoid

Features

- The clinical features are dependent both on the underlying cause and also on the rate of development of hyponatraemia. They may develop once the sodium reaches 115 mmol/L or may occur earlier if the fall is rapid. Values of 100 mmol/L or less are life threatening.

- The features of excess water are mainly neurological because of brain injury, and depend on the age of the patient and rate of development. They include confusion and headache, progressing to seizures and coma. In addition, in the hypervolaemic forms of excess water (where the fluid is confined to the ECF e.g. cardiac failure, nephrotic syndrome, and cirrhosis) oedema and fluid overload is apparent. In contrast, in the syndromes of excess water associated with SIADH the fluid is distributed throughout the ECF and ICF and there is no apparent fluid overload. In contrast, salt deficiency presents with features of hypovolaemia with tachycardia and postural hypotension.

Investigation

- Urinary sodium is very helpful in differentiating the underlying cause (Table 34.1).
- Assess volume status
- Other investigations as indicated e.g. serum and urine osmolality, cortisol, thyroid function, liver biochemistry.

Treatment

Salt deficiency (renal or non-renal)

- Increase dietary salt.
- May need intravenous normal saline if dehydrated

Excess water (cirrhosis, nephrotic syndrome, CCF)

- Fluid restriction to 500–1000 mL/24 h.
- Occasionally hypertonic (3%) saline (513 mmol/L) may be required in patients with acute symptomatic hyponatraemia. The appropriate infusion rate can be calculated from the formula:

  rate of sodium replacement (mmol/hour) = total body water (60% of body weight) × desired correction rate (0.5–1 mmol/h).

  E.g. for a 70 kg man:

  $Na^+ = 60\% \times 70$ kg $\times 1$ mmol/hr $= 42$ mmol/hr

  $$= 42 \times \frac{1000}{513} \qquad\qquad = 82 \text{ ml/hr of 3\% saline}$$

- Rapid normalization (faster than 0.5 mmol/h) of sodium may be associated with central pontine myelinolysis.

SIADH

See following chapter.

Chapter 35
Syndrome of inappropriate ADH

SIADH is a common cause of hyponatraemia. It is clinically normo-volaemic hyponatraemia, since the increased water is distributed through all compartments.

Criteria for diagnosis

- Hyponatraemia and hypotonic plasma (osmolality <270 mOsm/kg).
- Inappropriate urine osmolality >100 mOsm/kg.
- Excessive renal sodium loss (>20 mmol/L, often >50 mmol/L).
- Absence of clinical evidence of hypovolaemia or of volume over-load.
- Normal renal, adrenal, and thyroid function.
- NB Fluid restriction may reduce sodium loss
- Exclude adrenal or thyroid dysfunction.

Types of SIADH

Type 1
- erratic excess ADH secretion, unrelated to plasma osmolality commonest (40%) associated (not exclusively) with tumours.

Type 2
- 'reset osmostat': patients autoregulate around a lower serum osmolality
- chest and CNS disease.

Type 3
- 'leaky osmostat' normal osmoregulation until plasma hypotonicity develops when vasopressin secretion continues.

Type 4
- normal osmoregulated vasopressin secretion, possible receptor defect or alternative antidiuretic hormone.

Table 35.1 Causes of SIADH

Tumours	Small cell lung carcinoma, thymoma, lymphoma, leukaemia, sarcoma, mesothelioma
Chest disease	Infections (pneumonia, tuberculosis, empyema)
	Pneumothorax
	Asthma
	Positive pressure ventilation
CNS disorders	Infections (meningitis, encephalitis, abscess)
	Head injury
	Guillain Barré
	Vascular disorders (subarachnoid haemorrhage, cerebral thrombosis)
	Psychosis
Drugs	Chemotherapy (vincristine, vinblastine, cyclophosphamide)
	Psychiatric drugs (phenothiazines, MAOI)
	Carbamazepine
	Clofibrate
	Chlorpropamide
Metabolic	Hypothyroidism
	Glucocorticoid deficiency
	Acute intermittent porphyria
Idiopathic	

Treatment

- Treatment of the underlying cause.
- Fluid restriction to 500–1000 mL/24 h.
- If the problem is not temporary and fluid restriction long-term can be difficult for the patient, drug treatment may be tried. *Demeclocycline* may be effective by inducing partial nephrogenic DI. New specific vasopressin antagonists are under trial.
- In an emergency, saline infusion may be required – great care is required as rapid overcorrection of hyponatraemia may cause central pontine myelinolysis (demyelination). This can be avoided if the rate of correction does not exceed 0.5 mmol/L per hour (see p. 241).

Chapter 36
Hypothalamus

Pathophysiology

- The hypothalamus releases hormones that act as releasing hormones at the anterior pituitary gland. It also produces dopamine that inhibits PRL release from the anterior pituitary gland. It also synthesizes arginine vasopressin and oxytocin (see p. 228).
- The commonest syndrome to be associated with the hypothalamus is abnormal GnRH secretion leading to reduced gonadotrophin secretion and hypogonadism. Common causes are stress, weight loss, and excessive exercise. Management involves treatment of the cause if possible. Administration of pulsatile GnRH is usually effective at reversing the abnormality but rarely undertaken.

Hypothalamic syndrome

Uncommon but may occur due to a large tumour, following surgery for a craniopharyngioma, or due to infiltration from e.g. Langerhans cell histiocytosis. The typical features are hyperphagia and weight gain, loss of thirst sensation, DI, somnolence and behaviour change. Management can be challenging. E.g. DI with the loss of thirst sensation may require the prescription of regular fluid in addition to desmopressin, and monitoring with daily weights and fluid balance as a routine.

Metabolic effects of hypothalamic mass lesions

- appetite
  - hyperphagia and obesity
  - anorexia
- thirst
  - adipsia
  - compulsive drinking
- temperature
  - hyperthermia
  - hypothermia
- somnolence and coma.

Chapter 37
Eating disorders

Anorexia nervosa

Features

- Typical presentation is a woman aged <25 with weight loss, amenorrhoea, and behavioural changes.
- There is a long-term risk of severe osteoporosis associated with >6 months amenorrhoea. There is loss of bone mineral content and bone density with little or no recovery after resolution of the amenorrhoea.

Endocrine abnormalities

- Deficiency of GnRH, low LH and FSH, normal PRL, and low oestrogen in women or testosterone in men.
- Elevated circulating cortisol (usually non-suppressible with dexamethasone).
- Low normal thyroxine, reduced T_3, and normal TSH.
- Elevated resting GH levels.
- In addition, it is common to find various metabolic abnormalities such as reduced magnesium, zinc, phosphorus, and calcium levels in addition to hyponatraemia and hypokalaemia.
- Weight gain leads to a reversion of the prepubertal LH secretory pattern to the adult-like secretion. Administration of GnRH in a pulsatile pattern leads to normalization of the pituitary–gonadal axis, demonstrating that the primary abnormality is hypothalamic.

Management

The long-term treatment of these patients involves treatment of the underlying condition and then management of osteoporosis, although many patients will refuse oestrogen replacement.

Bulimia

Features

• Typically occurs in women who are slightly older than the group with anorexia nervosa. Weight may be normal and patients often deny the abnormal eating behaviour. Patients gorge themselves, using artificial means of avoiding excessive weight gain (laxatives, diuretic abuse, vomiting). This may be a cause of 'occult' hypo-kalaemia.

• These patients may or may not have menstrual irregularity. If menstrual irregularity is present, this is often associated with inadequate oestrogen secretion and anovulation.

Chapter 38
Pineal gland

Physiology

- The pineal gland lies behind the third ventricle, is highly vascular, and produces melatonin and other peptides.
- During daylight, light-induced hyperpolarization of the retinal photoreceptors inhibits signalling and the pineal gland is quiescent.
- Darkness stimulates the gland, and there is synthesis and release of melatonin.
- Melatonin levels are usually low during the day, rise during the evening, peak at midnight and then decline independent of sleep.
- Exposure to darkness during the day does not increase melatonin secretion.

Jet lag

- It is claimed that pharmacological doses of melatonin can reset the body clock.
- Studies have suggested that melatonin may reduce the severity or duration of jet lag. There are few safety data, and currently melatonin does not have a product licence in the UK.

Pineal and intracranial germ cell tumours

- *Incidence* 0.5%–3% intracranial neoplasms.
- *Epidemiology* M > F. All ages. 2/3 present between age 10 and 21 years.
- Germ cell tumours are now classified as germinomas or non-germinomatous germ cell tumours (choriocarcinoma, teratoma). The latter term includes the tumours previously called 'true' pinealomas.

Features

- raised intracranial pressure (compression of cerebral aqueduct), headache, and lethargy
- visual disturbance (pressure on quadrigeminal plate)
- Parinaud's syndrome (paralysis of upward gaze, convergent nystagmus, Argyll–Robertson pupils)
- ataxia
- pyramidal signs
- hypopituitarism
- DI
- sexual precocity in boys (excess hCG secretion mimics LH leading to Leydig cell testosterone secretion, or related to space-occupying mass).

Investigations

• imaging of craniospinal axis MRI/CT (may detect second tumour/metastases)
• CSF examination
• tumour markers (hCG, α-fetoprotein)
• cytology
• biopsy if tumour markers unhelpful
• pituitary function assessment.

Management

• External beam radiotherapy – standard therapy is to irradiate the whole craniospinal axis
• Germinomas are exquisitely radiosensitive.
• Chemotherapy may be indicated, e.g. vincristine, etopside, carboplatin.
• Recent work suggests that a combination of radiotherapy and chemotherapy can considerably increase long-term cure rates.

Prognosis

Excellent for germinomas (70–85% 5 year survival), but non-germinomatous germ cell tumours have a worse prognosis (15–40% 5 year survival).

Part III
Adrenal glands

Chapter 39
Anatomy and physiology

Anatomy

The normal adrenal glands weigh 4–5 g. The cortex represents 90% of the normal gland and surrounds the medulla. The arterial blood supply arises from the renal arteries, aorta, and inferior phrenic artery. Venous drainage occurs via the central vein into the inferior vena cava on the right, and into the left renal vein on the left.

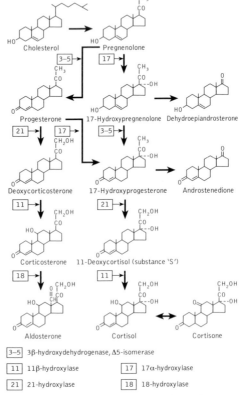

Fig 39.1 Pathways and enzymes involved in synthesis of glucocorticoids, mineralocorticoids, and adrenal androgens from a cholesterol precursor. © Reprinted from Besser & Thorner: *Clinical endocrinology*, by permission of the publisher Mosby.

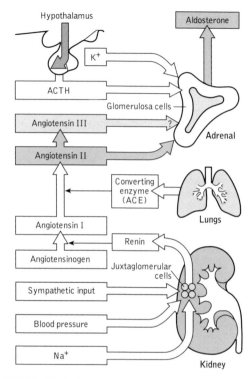

Fig. 39.2 Physiological mechanisms governing the production and secretion of aldosterone. © Reprinted from Besser & Thorner: *Clinical endocrinology*, by permission of the publisher Mosby.

Physiology

Glucocorticoids

Glucocorticoid (cortisol 10–20 mg/d) production occurs from the zona fasiculata and adrenal androgens arise form the zona reticularis. Both of these are under control of ACTH, which regulates both steroid synthesis, and also adrenocortical growth.

Mineralocorticoids

Mineralocorticoid (aldosterone 100–150 μg/d) synthesis occurs predominantly under the control of the renin–angiotensin system, in the zona glomerulosa and only 5–10% is under ACTH regulation.

Androgens

The adrenal gland also produces sex steroids, in the form of dehydroepiandrostenedione (DHEA) and androstenedione. The synthetic pathway is under the control of ACTH.

Chapter 40
Imaging

Computed tomography scanning

CT is the most widely used modality for imaging the adrenal glands. It is able to detect masses >5 mm in diameter, and is currently the optimal means of differentiating between different adrenal cortical pathologies.

Magnetic resonance imaging

MRI can also reliably detect adrenal masses >5–10 mm in diameter, and in some circumstances provides additional information to CT, e.g. differentiation of cortical from medullary tumours

Ultrasound imaging

Ultrasound detects masses >20 mm in diameter, but normal adrenal glands are not usually visible except in children. Body morphology and bowel gas can provide technical difficulties.

Further reading

Peppercorn PD, Grossman AB, Reznek RH. Imaging of incidentally discovered adrenal masses *Clinical Endocrinology* 1998; 48: 379–388.
Reznek RH, Armstrong P. The adrenal gland. *Clinical Endocrinology* 1994; 40: 561–576.

Normal adrenal

Normal adrenal cortex is assessed by measuring limb thickness, and is considered enlarged at >5 mm approximately the thickness of the diaphragmatic crus nearby.

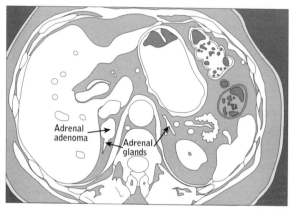

Fig. 40.1 Typical appearance of adrenal adenoma on CT scan.

Radionucleotide imaging

- *^{75}Se 6β-selenomethyl-19-norcholesterol* This isotope is concentrated in functioning steroid synthesizing tissue, and is used to image the adrenal cortex. It is particularly useful in determining whether a nodule is functioning or not. In addition it can be helpful in localizing residual adrenal tissue following failed bilateral adrenalectomy.

- *^{123}Iodine-metaiodobenzylguanidine* (MIBG) is a guanethidine analogue, concentrated in some phaeochromocytomas, paragangliomas, carcinoid tumours, and neuroblastomas, and is useful diagnostically. A different isotope, ^{131}I-MIBG, may be used therapeutically, e.g. in malignant phaeochromocytomas when the diagnostic imaging shows uptake.

Venous sampling

Adrenal vein sampling can be useful to lateralize an adenoma, or to differentiate an adenoma from bilateral hyperplasia. It is technically difficult – particularly catheterizing the right adrenal vein because of its drainage into the IVC. It may also be used to confirm the diagnosis of bilateral phaeochromocytoma.

Chapter 41
Mineralocorticoid excess

Definitions

The majority of cases of mineralocorticoid excess are due to excess aldosterone production which may be primary or secondary and are typically associated with hypertension and hypokalaemia.

• *Primary hyperaldosteronism* is a disorder of autonomous aldosterone hypersecretion with suppressed renin levels.

• *Secondary hyperaldosteronism* occurs when aldosterone hypersecretion occurs secondary to elevated circulating renin levels, due to renal artery stenosis, or renal hypoperfusion, and occasionally a very rare renin-producing tumour (reninoma).

• Other mineralocorticoids may occasionally be the cause of this syndrome (see opposite).

Causes of mineralocorticoid excess

Primary hyperaldosteronism

- Conn's syndrome (aldosterone-producing adrenal adenoma)
- bilateral adrenal hyperplasia
- glucocorticoid suppressible hyperaldosteronism
- aldosterone-producing adrenal carcinoma.

Secondary hyperaldosteronism

- renal artery stenosis
- renal hypoperfusion
- cirrhosis
- congestive cardiac failure
- nephrotic syndrome
- renin-secreting tumour.

Other mineralocorticoid excess syndromes

- apparent mineralocorticoid excess
- liquorice ingestion
- deoxycorticosterone and corticosterone
- ectopic ACTH secretion
- congenital adrenal hyperplasia
- exogenous mineralocorticoids.

'Pseudoaldosteronism' due to abnormal renal tubular transport

- Bartter's syndrome (p. 301)
- Gitelman's syndrome (p. 302)
- Liddle's syndrome (p. 300)

Chapter 42
Primary aldosteronism

Epidemiology

Primary hyperaldosteronism accounts for at least 2% (and possibly up to 10%) of hypertensive patients. The most common cause is a unilateral adrenal adenoma (see Table 42.1).

Pathophysiology

Aldosterone causes renal sodium retention and potassium loss. This results in expansion of body sodium content, resulting in suppression of renal renin synthesis. The direct action of aldosterone on the distal nephron causes sodium retention and loss of hydrogen and potassium ions, resulting in a hypokalaemic alkalosis, although serum potassium may not be significantly reduced and may be normal in up to 50% of cases.

Clinical features

- Moderately severe hypertension, which is often resistant to conventional therapy.
- Hypokalaemia is usually asymptomatic. Occasionally patients may present with tetany, myopathy, polyuria and nocturia (hypokalaemic nephrogenic diabetes insipidus) due to severe hypokalaemia.

Table 42.1 Causes of primary hyperaldosteronism

Condition	Relative frequency	Age	Sex	Pathology
Aldosteronoma (Conn's adenoma)	70%	3rd–6th decade	Predominant in females	Benign, adenoma, <2.5 cm diameter, yellow because of high cholesterol content
Idiopathic aldosteronism/ adrenal hyperplasia	Common	Older than Conn's	No sex difference	Macronodular or micronodular hyperplasia
Adrenal carcinoma	Rare	5th–7th decade (occasionally young)	More common in females	Tumour >4 cm in diameter – often larger, may be evidence of local invasion
Glucocorticoid suppressible hyperaldosteronism	Rare	Childhood	No sex difference	Bilateral hyperplasia of zona glomerulosa

Conn's syndrome – aldosterone-producing adenoma

Very high levels of aldosterone synthase are expressed, and greater amounts of aldosterone are usually produced than in other causes. Although aldosterone production is autonomous, ACTH has a greater stimulatory effect than angiotensin II, although a subtype that remain more responsive to angiotensin II has been described (implications for postural testing – see later).

Bilateral adrenal hyperplasia (bilateral idiopathic hyperaldosteronism)

This is the second most common form of primary hyperaldosteronism in adults. Hyperplasia is more commonly bilateral than unilateral, and may be associated with micronodular or macronodular hyperplasia. The pathophysiology is not known although aldosterone secretion is very sensitive to circulating angiotensin II, and not ACTH. Hypokalaemia tends to be milder.

Glucocorticoid-suppressible hyperaldosteronism (GSH)

A rare autosomal dominantly inherited condition due to the presence of a chimeric gene (8q22) containing the 5′ sequence which determines regulation of the 11β-hydroxylase gene (*CYP11B1*) coding for the enzyme catalysing the last step in cortisol synthesis, and the 3′ sequence from the aldosterone synthase gene (*CYP11B2*) coding for the enzyme catalysing the last step in aldosterone synthesis. This results in expression of aldosterone synthase in the zona fasiculata as well as the zona glomerulosa and aldosterone secretion becomes under ACTH control. Glucocorticoids lead to suppression of ACTH and suppression of aldosterone production.

Early haemorrhagic strokes are characteristic in GSH pedigrees.

Aldosterone-producing carcinoma

Rare, and usually associated with excessive secretion of other corticosteroids (cortisol, androgen, oestrogen). Hypokalaemia may be profound, and aldosterone levels very high.

Investigation

- NB If serum potassium is <3 mmol/L, this should be normalized before measuring aldosterone.
- Many antihypertensive drugs interfere with testing (see Table 2). *α*-Blockers, e.g. doxazosin may be used if continued treatment is required.

Screening

Who?

- Patients resistant to conventional antihypertensive medication
- Hypertension associated with hypokalaemia
- Hypertension developing before age of 40 years.

How?

- *Serum potassium* Hypokalaemic alkalosis is highly suggestive of primary hyperaldosteronism, but 20–40% patients may be normokalaemic. A low salt diet will often mask hypokalaemia.
- *Urinary potassium* excretion>30 mmol/24 h following discontinuation of diuretics, in the presence of hypokalaemia, is suggestive of hyperaldosteronism.
- *Plasma renin* Suppressed in patients with primary hyperaldosteronism, but also suppressed in a third of patients with essential hypertension. Sodium intake and antihypertensive medication may alter plasma renin levels (see Table 42.3).
- *Aldosterone: renin ratio* A high ratio is suggestive of primary hyperaldosteronism (aldosterone [pmol/L]/plasma renin activity [ng/mL/h] >750 or aldosterone [ng/dl]/plasma renin activity [ng/mL/h] >30–50). The greater the ratio, the more likely the diagnosis of primary aldosteronism. The timing (morning), posture (upright), potassium (normal) and concomitant medication (avoid antihypertensive agents in particular *β*-blockers and diuretics) interfering with renin and aldosterone (Table 2), should be standardized. A false negative is found in patients with chronic renal failure.

Table 42.2 Drugs and investigation of renin–angiotensin II axis

Drug	Effect	Duration of washout required (weeks)
ACE inhibitors and angiotensin II antagonists	↑ PRA	2
Diuretics	↑ PRA	2
Spironolactone	↑ PRA	6
β-blockers	↓ PRA	2
Calcium channel blockers	↓ Aldosterone	2

Confirmation of hyperaldosteronism and differentiation of underlying cause

- *Oral salt loading* A high sodium diet (120 mmol sodium/day) for 3 days may precipitate hypokalaemia in a patients with normokalaemia on a low salt diet. In addition, since the normal response to a salt load is aldosterone suppression, the lack of suppression in primary hyperaldosteronism can be used to confirm the diagnosis. Correct hypokalaemia before measuring aldosterone levels, as low potassium levels will tend to suppress aldosterone *per se*.

- *Postural test* Plasma aldosterone, renin, and cortisol are measured after the patient has been lying down overnight, and repeated after an upright posture has been maintained for 4 h. This test relies on the fact that aldosterone production from the majority of adenomas is dependent on ACTH secretion, but independent of posture, whereas in adrenal hyperplasia, aldosterone production is stimulated by angiotensin II in response to an upright posture. Failure of aldosterone to rise to more than a third above baseline is suggestive of an adenoma.

- *Serum cortisol* is measured to confirm the circadian pattern of ACTH secretion with a fall in cortisol after 4 h. A rise in the post-ambulatory cortisol invalidates the test.

- *Urinary 18 hydroxycortisol* Elevated levels of this precursor are found in primary aldosteronism due to a Conn's adenoma or glucocorticoid suppressible hyperaldosteronism. (GSH >> Conn's > adrenal hyperplasia)

- *Dexamethasone suppression test* Treatment with dexamethasone (0.5 mg 6 hourly) for >3 days leads to lowering of aldosterone and blood pressure in glucocorticoid suppressible hyperaldosteronism.

- *Genetic analysis* Can be used to confirm the diagnosis of glucocorticoid suppressible hypertension.

- *Other dynamic tests* which may be helpful include the response to an ACEI which may help differentiate adenomas from hyperplasia. Plasma aldosterone is measured in the sitting position, basally and 60 min after captopril. Inhibition of angiotensin II leads to a fall in aldosterone in patients with idiopathic hyperaldosteronism but not in Conn's syndrome. Another test which is rarely used is the fludrocortisone suppression test where fludrocortisone 400 μg/d for 4 days leads to no suppression of aldosterone in Conn's syndrome.

Table 42.3 Differential diagnosis of primary hyperaldosteronism

Test		Upright posture and time	ACE inhibitor	Dexamethasone suppression
Normal	PRA	↑	↑	→
	Aldosterone	↑	↓	→
Aldosterone-producing adenoma	PRA	→	→	→
	Aldosterone	↓	→	→
Angiotensin-responsive adenoma (?~20% adenomas)	PRA	↑	↑	→
	Aldosterone	↑	↓	→
Idiopathic adrenal hyperplasia	PRA	↑	↑	→
	Aldosterone	↑	↓	→
Glucocorticoid-suppressible hyperaldosteronism	PRA	→	→	↑
	Aldosterone	↓	→	↓

Localization

CT/MRI scan

- Identifies most adenomas >5 mm diameter. Bilateral abnormalities or tumours <1 cm in diameter require further localization procedures.
- In idiopathic aldosteronism, both glands appear enlarged or normal in size.
- Macronodular hyperplasia may result in identifiable nodules on imaging.
- A mass >4 cm in size is suspicious of carcinoma but is unusual in Conn's syndrome.
- NB. In essential hypertension nodules are described.

Adrenal vein sampling

Aldosterone measurements from both adrenal veins allow a gradient between the two sides to be identified in the case of unilateral disease. It is the gold standard for differentiation between uni- and bilateral aldosterone production, but cannulating the right adrenal vein is technically difficult. Cortisol measurements should also be taken concomitantly with aldosterone, to confirm successful positioning within the adrenal veins.

Radiolabelled iodocholesterol scanning

Unilateral increase uptake indicates the presence of an adenoma. Prior administration of dexamethasone (e.g. 1 mg 4× daily for 3 days before isotope administration and for 1 week afterwards) to suppress cortisol production increases accuracy. Normal adrenal is not visualized before the 5th day using the dexamethasone protocol, and adenomas are seen before this.

Treatment

Surgery

Adrenalectomy is the treatment of choice for aldosterone secreting adenomas. Hypertension is cured in about 70%. If it persists (more likely in those with long-standing hypertension and old people) it is more amenable to medical treatment. The blood pressure response to treatment with spironolactone (200–400 mg/d) before surgery can be used to predict the response to surgery of patients with adenomas. (NB Spironolactone has a long half-life and may need to be stopped for 2 days before surgery to avoid postoperative mineralocorticoid deficiency). Overall 50% become normotensive in 1 month and 70% within 1 year.

Laparoscopic adrenalectomy is increasingly being successfully performed and is associated with lower morbidity and promising results. Presurgical spironolactone treatment may be used to correct potassium stores before surgery.

Angiotensin II responsive adenomas can be successfully treated with surgery, but may also respond to ACEI.

Surgery is contra-indicated in patients with idiopathic hyperaldosteronism as even bilateral adrenalectomy does not cure the hypertension.

Medical treatment

The aldosterone antagonist *spironolactone* (200–400 mg/day) has been used successfully for many years to treat the hypertension and hypokalaemia associated with bilateral adrenal hyperplasia and idiopathic hyperaldosteronism. There may be a delay in response of hypertension of 4–8 weeks. However, combination with other antihypertensive agents (ACEI and calcium channel blockers) is usually required. Side-effects are common – particularly gynaecomastia and impotence in men, menstrual irregularities in women, and gastrointestinal effects.

Alternative drugs include the potassium-sparing diuretics *amiloride* and *triamterene*. Calcium channel antagonists may also be helpful.

Glucocorticoid-suppressible hyperaldosteronism can be treated with low dose *dexamethasone* (0.5 mg on going to bed and 0.25 mg on waking). Side-effects often limit therapy, and spironolactone treatment is often preferred. In addition, spironolactone may reduce the poorly understood increased risk of stroke in this group.

Adrenal carcinoma

Surgery and postoperative adrenolytic therapy with *ortho-para*-DDD (*mitotane*) is usually required, but the prognosis is usually poor (see p. 292).

Further reading

Ganguly A. Primary aldosteronism. *New England Journal of Medicine* 1998; 339: 1828–1833.

Chapter 43
Excess other mineralocorticoids

Epidemiology

Occasionally, the clinical syndrome of hyperaldosteronism is not associated with excess aldosterone, and a process due to another mineralocorticoid is suspected. These conditions are rare.

When to suspect it?

Hypertension and hypokalaemic alkalosis in association with low plasma renin activity and the absence of elevated aldosterone.

Apparent mineralocorticoid excess

This is due to deficiency of the 11β-hydroxysteroid dehydrogenase (HSD) enzyme type 2, which usually protects the distal nephron mineralocorticoid receptor from stimulation by cortisol. The mineralocorticoid receptor has an equal affinity for cortisol and aldosterone, but there is a 100-fold excess of circulating cortisol over aldosterone. Cortisol is metabolized to the relatively inactive cortisone by 11βHSD at the mineralocorticoid receptor.

Congenital absence of the enzyme or inhibition of its activity (e.g. following liquorice ingestion) allows cortisol to stimulate the receptor and leads to severe hypertension. This condition is seen predominantly in children, presenting with failure to thrive, thirst, polyuria, and severe hypertension. Patients are not cushingoid as there is intact negative feedback.

Biochemistry

• Suppression of PRA and aldosterone
• Elevated ratio of urinary tetrahydrocortisol and *allo*-tetrahydrocortisol to tetrahydrocortisone (>10 in AME; normal = 1).

Treatment

Dexamethasone leads to suppression of ACTH secretion, reduced cortisol concentrations, and lowered blood pressure. It has a much lower affinity for the mineralocorticoid receptor.

Deoxycorticosterone and corticosterone

Two forms of congenital adrenal hyperplasia (see p. 368) are associated with this syndrome:

- 17α-hydroxylase deficiency (deoxycorticosterone and corticosterone)
- 11β-hydroxylase (deoxycorticosterone)

Glucocorticoid replacement to inhibit ACTH is effective treatment for these conditions.

Adrenal tumours rarely secrete excessive amounts of deoxycorticosterone or corticosterone. Usually this is concomitant with excessive aldosterone production, but occasionally it may occur in an isolated fashion.

Ectopic ACTH syndrome

The aldosterone receptor has equal affinity for cortisol and aldosterone, and is usually protected from the effects of stimulation by cortisol by the 11β-hydroxysteroid type 2 dehydrogenase enzyme which converts cortisol to cortisone to protect the receptor. In the syndrome of ectopic ACTH, this protection is overcome because of high cortisol secretion rates which saturate the enzyme, leading to impaired conversion of cortisol to cortisone, and thus hypokalaemia and hypertension.

Further reading

Chidiac RM, Aron DC. Incidentalomas. *Endocrinology and Metabolism Clinics of North America* 1997;26: 233–253.

Kloos RT, Gross MD, Francis IR, Korobkin M, Shapiro B. Incidentally discovered adrenal masses. *Endocrine Reviews* 1995;16: 460–484.

Newell-Price J, Grossman A. Adrenal incidentaloma. *Postgraduate Medical Journal* 1996;72: 207–210.

Turner HE, Moore NR, Byrne JV, Wass JAH. Pituitary, adrenal and thyroid incidentalomas *Endocrin Related Cancer* 1998;5: 131–150.

Chapter 44
Adrenal Cushing's syndrome

Definition and epidemiology

• Cushing's syndrome results from chronic excess cortisol, and is described on page 158.

• The causes may be classified as ACTH dependent and ACTH independent. This section describes ACTH-independent Cushing's syndrome, which is due to adrenal tumours (benign and malignant), and is responsible for 10–20% cases of Cushing's syndrome.

• Adrenal tumours causing Cushing's syndrome are commoner in women. The peak incidence is in the fourth and fifth decade.

• Causes and relative frequencies of adrenal Cushing's syndrome in adults:
  – adrenal adenoma   10%
  – adrenal carcinoma   8%
  – bilateral micronodular adrenal hyperplasia   1%
  – bilateral macronodular hyperplasia   1%

Pathophysiology

• Benign adenomas are usually encapsulated, and <6 cm in diameter. They are usually associated with pure glucocorticoid excess.

• Adrenal carcinomas are usually >6 cm in diameter, although they may be smaller, and are often associated with local invasion and metastases at the time of diagnosis. They may be associated with secretion of excess androgen production in addition to cortisol. Occasionally they may be associated with mineralocorticoid or oestrogen secretion.

• Adrenal hyperplasia may be micronodular (<1 cm diameter) or macronodular (>1 cm). A rare cause of adrenal hyperplasia causing Cushing's syndrome due to inappropriate adrenal responsiveness to gastric inhibitory peptide (GIP) has been reported, resulting in food-induced glucocorticoid excess.

• *Carney complex* (see p. 731) is an autosomal dominant condition characterized by atrial myxomas, spotty skin pigmentation, peripheral nerve tumours, and endocrine disorders e.g. Cushing's syndrome due to pigmented adrenal nodular hyperplasia.

Clinical features

- The clinical features of ACTH independent Cushing's syndrome are as described on p. 161 in the section on ACTH-dependent disease.

- It is important to note that in patients with adrenal carcinoma, there may also be features related to excessive androgen production in women, and also a relatively more rapid time course of development of the syndrome.

Investigation

- Once the presence of Cushing's syndrome is confirmed (page 162), subsequent investigation of the cause depends on whether ACTH is suppressed (ACTH independent) or measurable/elevated (ACTH dependent) – see page 164.

- Patients with ACTH-independent Cushing's syndrome do not suppress cortisol to <50% basal on high dose dexamethasone testing, and fail to show a rise in cortisol and ACTH following administration of CRH. (The latter test is often important when patients have borderline/low ACTH to differentiate pituitary dependent disease from adrenal.)

- ACTH-independent causes are adrenal in origin, and the mainstay of further investigation is adrenal imaging.

- CT scan allows excellent visualization of the adrenal glands and their anatomy.

- Adenomas are usually small and homogeneous, and usually associated with contralateral gland atrophy.

- Adrenal carcinomas are usually >6 cm in diameter, heterogeneous with calcification and necrosis, and evidence of local invasion.

Treatment (see also p. 168)

Adrenal adenoma

- Unilateral adrenalectomy (laparoscopic or open) is curative.
- Postoperative temporary adrenal insufficiency ensues because of long-term suppression of ACTH and the contralateral adrenal gland, requiring glucocorticoid replacement for up to 2 years.

Adrenal carcinoma

- Surgery is useful to debulk tumour mass, and occasionally adrenalectomy and local clearance leads to cure. However, most patients have distant metastases at the time of diagnosis.
- Postoperative drug treatment with the adrenolytic agent *mitotane* (*ortho-para* DDD) 3–12 g daily is usually used. This may lead to adrenal insufficiency and glucocorticoid replacement may be required. Side-effects may limit therapy – nausea and vomiting, dizziness, and diarrhoea. Monitoring of drug levels can be helpful to ensure concentrations within the therapeutic range (14–20 μg/mL), and so limit unwanted side-effects.
- Other drugs may be required to control cortisol hypersecretion (*metyrapone, aminoglutethamide*).
- Newer treatments such as *suramin, 5-fluorouracil,* and *gossypol* have also been tried.

Bilateral adrenal hyperplasia

Bilateral adrenalectomy is curative. Lifelong glucocorticoid and mineralocorticoid treatment is required.

Prognosis

- Adrenal adenomas which are successfully treated with surgery have a good prognosis, and recurrence is unlikely. The prognosis depends on the long-term effects of excess cortisol before treatment – in particular atherosclerosis and osteoporosis.

- The prognosis for adrenal carcinoma is very poor, despite surgery. Reports suggest a 5 year survival of 22%, and median survival time of 14 months. Age >40 years and distant metastases are associated with a worse prognosis.

Subclinical Cushing's syndrome

- Describes the subset of patients with apparently silent adrenal cortical adenomas that possess some features of autonomous function.

- Cortisol secretion may be sufficient to suppress ACTH and suppress contralateral adrenal function.

- There may be subtle changes in cortisol secretion with loss of normal diurnal rhythm of cortisol secretion and failure of dexamethasone suppressibility despite apparently normal cortisol levels.

- At present it is not clear whether these changes are associated with clinically relevant symptomatology. There have been suggestions that these patients may have a higher prevalence of diabetes, hypertension, and osteoporosis.

- The natural history of this condition remains to be determined.

Chapter 45
Adrenal surgery

Adrenalectomy

Open adrenalectomy has been the standard approach for all adrenal pathology. More recently the advent of the laparoscopic approach has led to open surgery being reserved in many centres for either larger lesions (>6 cm), or suspected malignancy.

Laparoscopic adrenalectomy

First performed in 1992, this procedure has become the procedure of choice in many centres for removal of most adrenal tumours. There have been to date, no prospective randomized clinical trials, but retrospective comparisons with open approaches suggest reduced hospital stay, reduced analgesic requirements and lower postoperative morbidity. However, there are few long-term outcome data on this technique. Cure rate and recurrence/regrowth due to incomplete excision or spillage will need to be assessed.

Currently it appears to be most useful in the management of small (<6 cm) benign adenomas. Larger tumours may be malignant and therefore should be operated on via an open incision, and bilateral adrenalectomy may be problematic because of longer operating times.

Further reading

Dudley NE, Harrison BJ. Comparison of open posterior versus transperitoneal laparoscopic adrenalectomy. *British Journal of Surgery* 1999; 86: 656–660.

Wells SA, Merke DP, Cutler GB, Norton JA, Lacroix A. The role of laparoscopic surgery in adrenal disease. *Journal of Clinical Endocrinology and Metabolism* 1998; 83: 3041–3049.

Preoperative preparation of patients

* Cushing's – metyrapone or ketoconazole (see p. 170)
* Phaeochromocytoma – α- and β-blockade (see p. 340).

Perioperative management of patients undergoing adrenalectomy

Adrenal cortical tumours (benign and malignant)/bilateral adrenalectomy for Cushing's syndrome

* Perioperative glucocorticoid cover is required, as even 'silent' adenomas may be associated with subclinical excess cortisol secretion and hence suppression of the contralateral adrenal gland.
* Hydrocortisone is given as for pituitary surgery – 100 mg i/m with the premedication, and then continued every 6 h for 24–48 h, until the patient can take oral medication and is eating and drinking.
* This is changed to oral hydrocortisone at double replacement dose – 20 mg on waking, 10 mg at lunchtime and 10 mg at 5 p.m., and mineralocorticoid replacement commenced if bilateral adrenalectomy has been performed (100 μg fludrocortisone daily). Electrolytes and blood pressure guide adequacy of treatment. Normal replacement hydrocortisone (10, 5, 5 mg) can be commenced when the patient is recovered and may be omitted altogether if the patient did not have preoperative evidence of Cushing's syndrome/suppression of the contralateral gland/bilateral adrenalectomy. Mineralocorticoid replacement is only required in patients who have had bilateral adrenalectomy.
* A short synacthen test (off hydrocortisone for at least 24 h) is performed after at least 2 weeks to demonstrate adequate function of the contralateral adrenal. However, in patients with ACTH-independent Cushing's syndrome, it may take up to 2 years for full recovery of the contralateral adrenal gland to recover.
* The exception is patients undergoing adrenalectomy for mineralocorticoid-secreting tumour. These patients do not usually require peroperative glucocorticoid replacement, but preoperative amiloride or spironolactone allows recovery of potassium stores and control of hypertension prior to surgery.

Chapter 46

Renal tubular
abnormalities

Background

Bartter's syndrome and Gitelman's syndrome are both associated with hypokalaemic alkalosis and activation of the renin–angiotensin system, but in the absence of hypertension. In contrast, Liddle's syndrome is associated with hypokalaemic alkalosis and hypertension but low renin and aldosterone levels.

Liddle's syndrome

A rare autosomal dominant (AD) condition with variable penetrance. Mutations have been localized to genes on chromosome 16.

Cause

A mutation in the gene encoding the ß or γ subunit of the highly selective epithelial sodium channel in the distal nephron. This leads to constitutive activation of sodium/potassium exchange independent of circulating mineralocorticoid.

Features

Hypokalaemia and hypertension

Investigation

• hypokalaemic alkalosis
• suppressed renin and aldosterone levels

Treatment

Hypertension responds to amiloride but not spironolactone, because amiloride acts on the sodium channel directly whereas spironolactone acts on the mineralocorticoid receptor.

Bartter's syndrome

Cause

Loss of function of the bumetanide-sensitive Na–K–2Cl co-transporter in the thick ascending limb of the loop of Henle. Linkage of the disease has been shown to 15q15–q21. Inactivation of the co-transporter leads to salt wasting, activation of the renin–angiotensin system, and increased aldosterone which leads to increased sodium reabsorption at the distal nephron and causes hypokalaemic alkalosis. Reabsorption of calcium also occurs in the thick ascending loop and thus inactivation leads to hypercalciuria. Mutations in the rat outer medullary K channel (*ROMK*) gene have also been shown in some families, leading to the same clinical syndrome. The lack of associated hypertension is thought to be due to increased prostaglandin production from the renal medullary interstitial tissue in response to hypokalaemia.

- Rare (~1/million) autosomal recessive hypokalaemic metabolic alkalosis associated with salt wasting and normal or reduced blood pressure
- Usually present at an early age (<5 years).

Features

- intravascular volume depletion
- seizures
- tetany
- muscle weakness.

There is also an antenatal variant which is a life-threatening disorder of renal tubular hypokalaemic alkalosis and hypercalciuria.

Investigation

- hypokalaemic alkalosis
- increased PRA and aldosterone
- hypercalciuria

Treatment

- *Potassium replacement* Potassium sparing diuretics may be helpful. However, they are usually inadequate in correcting hypokalaemia. Prostaglandin synthase inhibitors (NSAIDS) e.g. indomethacin 2–5 mg/kg per day or ibuprofen may be required.
- ACEI in adults may be useful.

Gitelman's syndrome

Cause

• Loss of function in the thiazide-sensitive Na–Cl transporter of the distal convoluted tubule (DCT). Linkage to 16q13 has been shown. This leads to salt wasting, hypovolaemia, and metabolic alkalosis. Hypovolaemia leads to activation of the renin–angiotensin system, and increased aldosterone levels.

• Hypokalaemic alkalosis in conjunction with hypocalciuria and hypomagnaesaemia.

• Present at older ages without overt hypovolaemia (essentially a less severe phenotype of Bartter's syndrome).

Investigation

• hypokalaemic alkalosis, in association with increased renin and aldosterone

• hypomagnaesaemia

• hypocalciuria.

Treatment

• potassium and magnesium replacement.

• potassium sparing diuretics may be required.

Further reading

Amirlak I, Dawson KP. Bartter syndrome. *Quarterly Journal of Medicine* 2000; 93: 207–215.

Chapter 47
Mineralocorticoid deficiency

Epidemiology

Rare apart from the hyporeninaemic hypoaldosteronism associated with diabetes mellitus.

Causes

Congenital

- *Adrenal hypoplasia* (X-linked failure of development of the adrenal gland. Presents in infancy with salt losing state. Differentiated form CAH by normal external genitalia and steroid levels).
- *CAH* (certain types – most commonly 21-hydroxylase deficiency – are associated with MC deficiency; see p. 364).
- Rare *inherited disorders* of aldosterone biosynthesis.
- *Adrenoleukodystrophy* (X-linked affecting 1/20 000 males, where very long chain fatty acids cannot be oxidized in peroxisomes and accumulate in tissues.
- *Pseudohypoaldosteronism* (inherited resistance to the action of aldosterone, see p. 794). Autosomal dominant and recessive forms are described. Usually presents in infancy. Treated with sodium chloride.

Acquired

- *Adrenal insufficiency* (see p. 306).
- *Drugs* Heparin, cyclosporin (heparin for >5 days, may cause severe hyperkalaemia due to a toxic effect on the zona glomerulosa).
- *Hyporeninaemic hypoaldosteronism* Interference with the renin–angiotensin system leads to mineralocorticoid deficiency and hyperkalaemic acidosis (type IV renal tubular acidosis). e.g. diabetic nephropathy. Treatment is fludrocortisone and potassium restriction. ACEI may produce a similar biochemical picture, but here the PRA will be elevated as there is no angiotensin II feedback on renin.

Treatment

Fludrocortisone.

Chapter 48
Adrenal insufficiency

Definition

Adrenal insufficiency results from inadequate adrenocortical function, and may be due to destruction of the adrenal cortex (primary or Addison's disease), or due to disordered pituitary and hypothalamic function (secondary).

Epidemiology

- The incidence of Addison's disease is approximately 40–60/million adults.
- Secondary adrenal insufficiency is most commonly due to suppression of pituitary–hypothalamic function by exogenous glucocorticoid administration.

Causes of secondary adrenal insufficiency

Lesions of the hypothalamus and/or pituitary gland

* *tumours* pituitary tumour, metastases, craniopharyngioma
* *infection* tuberculosis
* *inflammation* sarcoidosis, histiocytosis X, haemochromatosis, lymphocytic hypophysitis
* *iatrogenic* surgery, radiotherapy
* *other* isolated ACTH deficiency, trauma.

Suppression of the hypothalamo–pituitary–adrenal axis

* glucocorticoid administration
* Cushing's disease (after pituitary tumour removal).

Features of secondary adrenal insufficiency

As primary (p. 312), except:
* absence of pigmentation – skin is pale
* absence of mineralocoticoid deficiency
* associated features of underlying cause, e.g. visual field defects if pituitary tumour
* other endocrine deficiencies may manifest due to pituitary failure (p. 116, Chapter 13))
* acute onset may occur due to pituitary apoplexy.

Isolated ACTH deficiency

* rare.
* pathogenesis unclear – may be autoimmune (associated with other autoimmune conditions, and antipituitary antibodies described in some patients).
* absent ACTH response to CRH.
* POMC mutations and POMC processing abnormalities (e.g. proconvertase PC1).

Pathophysiology

Primary

* Adrenal gland destruction or dysfunction occurs due to a disease process which usually involves all three zones of the adrenal cortex, resulting in inadequate glucocorticoid, mineralocorticoid, and androgen secretion. The manifestations of insufficiency do not usually appear till at least 90% of the gland has been destroyed, and are usually gradual in onset, with partial adrenal insufficiency leading to an impaired cortisol response to stress, and the features of complete insufficiency occurring later. Acute adrenal insufficiency may occur in the context of acute septicaemia (e.g. meningococcal or haemorrhage).

* Mineralocortcoid deficiency leads to reduced sodium retention and hypotension with reduced intravascular volume, in addition to hyperkalaemia due to reduced renal potassium and hydrogen ion excretion.

* Androgen deficiency presents in women with reduced axillary and pubic hair and reduced libido. (Testicular production of androgens is more important in males.)

* Lack of cortisol negative feedback increases CRH and ACTH secretion. An increase in other POMC-related peptides leads to skin pigmentation and other mucous membranes.

Secondary

* Inadequate ACTH results in deficient cortisol production (and reduced androgens in women).

* There is no pigmentation because ACTH and POMC secretion is reduced. Mineralocorticoid secretion remains normal as it is mainly regulated by the renin–angiotensin system.

* The onset is usually gradual with partial ACTH deficiency resulting in reduced response to stress. Prolonged ACTH deficiency leads to atrophy of the zona fasiculata and reduced ability to respond acutely to ACTH.

Investigation

See p. 117 for pituitary/hypothalamic disease and p. 324 for long-term endogenous or exogenous glucocorticoids.

Chapter 49
Addison's disease

Causes of primary adrenal insufficiency

- *Autoimmune* Commonest cause in developed world (approximately 70% cases)
- Autoimmune polyglandular deficiency type 1 or 2 (p. 313).
- *Malignancy* Metastatic (lung, breast, kidney – adrenal metastases found in ~50% of patients, but symptomatic adrenal insufficiency much less common), lymphoma.
- *Infiltration* amyloid, haemochromatosis.
- *Infection*
  - tuberculosis (medulla more frequently destroyed than cortex)
  - fungal e.g. histoplasmosis, cryptococcosis
  - opportunistic infections in e.g. AIDS – CMV, mycobacterium intracellulare, cryptococcus (up to 5% patients with AIDS develop primary adrenal insufficiency in the late stages).
- *Vascular* haemorrhage e.g. anticoagulants, Waterhouse–Friedrichson syndrome in meningococcal septicaemia.
- *Infarction* (e.g. secondary to thrombosis in antiphospholipid syndrome)
- *Adrenomyeloneuropathy* (X-linked recessive disorder of metabolism of fatty acids, leading to spastic paralysis and adrenal insufficiency. Onset early adulthood)
- *Adrenoleucodystrophy* (inherited disorder of fatty acid metabolism, presenting in childhood, and progressing to quadraparesis and dementia in association with adrenal failure)
- *CAH* (see p. 364).
- *Congenital adrenal hypoplasia* (rare familial failure of adrenal cortical development due to mutations/deletion of *DAX 1* gene)
- *Iatrogenic*
  - adrenalectomy
  - drugs: ketoconazole and fluconazole (inhibit cortisol synthesis), phenytoin, rifampicin (increases cortisol metabolism), etomidate, aminoglutethamide (usually do not cause hypoadrenalism unless reduced adrenal or pituitary reserve)

Autoimmune adrenalitis

- Mediated by humoral and cell-mediated immune mechanisms. Autoimmune insufficiency associated with polyglandular autoimmune syndrome is more common in females (70%).

- Adrenal cortex antibodies are present in the majority of patients at diagnosis, and although titres decline and eventually disappear, they are still found in approximately 70% of patients 10 years later. Up to 20% patients/year with positive adrenal antibodies develop adrenal insufficiency. Antibodies to 21-hydroxylase are commonly found, although the exact nature of other antibodies that block the effect of ACTH for example are yet to be elucidated.

- Antiadrenal antibodies are found in <2% of patients with other autoimmune endocrine disease (Hashimoto's thyroiditis, diabetes mellitus, autoimmune hypothyroidism, hypoparathyroidism, pernicious anaemia). In addition, antibodies to other endocrine glands are commonly found in patients with autoimmune adrenal insufficiency (thyroid microsomal in 50%, gastric parietal cell, parathyroid, and ovary and testis).

- Polyglandular autoimmune conditions (see p. 313). The presence of 17-hydroxylase antibodies in association with 21-hydroxylase antibodies is a good marker of patients at risk of developing premature ovarian failure in association with primary adrenal failure.

- Patients with type 1 diabetes mellitus and autoimmune thyroid disease only rarely develop autoimmune adrenal insufficiency. Approximately 50% of patients with Addison's disease have other autoimmune, or endocrine disorders.

Clinical features

Chronic

- anorexia and weight loss (>90%)
- tiredness
- weakness (generalized – no particular muscle groups)
- pigmentation (generalized, but most common in light exposed areas, and areas exposed to pressure (elbows and knees, and under bras and belts), mucosae and scars acquired after onset of adrenal insufficiency). Look at palmar creases in Caucasians.
- dizziness and postural hypotension
- gastrointestinal symptoms (nausea and vomiting, abdominal pain, diarrhoea)
- arthralgia and myalgia
- symptomatic hypoglycaemia (rare in adults)
- decreased axillary and pubic hair and reduced libido in women
- pyrexia of unknown origin (rarely)

Associated conditions

- vitiligo
- features of other autoimmune endocrinopathies.

Laboratory investigations

- hyponatraemia
- hyperkalaemia
- elevated urea
- anaemia (normocytic normochromic)
- elevated ESR
- eosinophilia
- mild hypercalcaemia.

Autoimmune polyglandular syndrome type 1

* autosomal recessive
* hypoparathyroidism (90%)
* chronic mucocutaneous candidiasis
* primary adrenal insufficiency (60%)
* primary gonadal failure
* primary hypothyroidism
* rarely hypopituitarism, diabetes insipidus
* associated malabsorption, pernicious anaemia, chronic active hepatitis, vitiligo.

Autoimmune polyglandular syndrome type 2

* autosomal recessive, autosomal dominant, polygenic
* adrenal insufficiency (100%)
* primary hypothyroidism
* type 1 diabetes mellitus
* primary gonadal failure
* rarely diabetes insipidus
* associated vitiligo, myasthenia gravis, alopecia, pernicious anaemia, immune thrombocytopenic purpura.

Investigation of primary adrenal insufficiency

Electrolytes

* hyponatraemia is present in 90% and hyperkalaemia in 65%
* elevated urea.

Serum cortisol and ACTH

* Undetectable serum cortisol is diagnostic of adrenal insufficiency, but the basal cortisol is usually in the normal range. A cortisol >580 nmol/L precludes the diagnosis. At times of acute stress, an inappropriately low cortisol is very suggestive of the diagnosis.
* Simultaneous 9 a.m. cortisol and ACTH will show an elevated ACTH for the level of cortisol. This is a very sensitive means of detecting Addison's disease.
* NB. Drugs causing increased cortisol-binding globulin (e.g. oestrogens) will result in higher total cortisol concentration measurements.

Response to ACTH

Short synacthen test

* Following basal cortisol measurement, 250 μg synacthen is administered i/m and serum cortisol checked at 30 and 60 min.
* Serum cortisol should rise to a peak of 580 nmol/L.
* Failure to respond suggests adrenal failure.
* A long synacthen test may be required to confirm secondary adrenal failure if ACTH is equivocal.
* Recent onset secondary adrenal failure (2 weeks) may produce a normal response to a short synacthen test.
* (There is recent interest in the low dose (1 μg ACTH) synacthen test as a more physiological assessment of adrenal reserve).

Long synacthen test

* Following basal cortisol level, depot synacthen 1 mg i/m is administered, and serum cortisol measured at 30, 60, 120 min, 4, 8, 12 and 24 h. A normal response is an elevation in serum cortisol to >1000 nmol/L.

Emergency management of acute adrenal insufficiency

- This is a life-threatening emergency, and should be treated if there is strong clinical suspicion rather than waiting for confirmatory test results.
- Blood should be taken for urgent analysis of electrolytes and glucose, in addition to cortisol and ACTH.

Fluids

Large volumes of 0.9% saline are required to reverse the volume depletion and sodium deficiency. Several litres may be required in the first 24–48 h.

Hydrocortisone

- A bolus dose of 100 mg hydrocortisone is administered intravenously. Hydrocortisone 100 mg i/m is then continued 6 hourly for 24–48 h, or until the patient can take oral therapy. Double replacement dose hydrocortisone (20, 10 and 10 mg orally) can then be instituted until well.
- Specific mineralocorticoid replacement is not required as the high dose glucocorticoid has sufficient mineralocorticoid effects. Once the dose of glucocorticoid is reduced after a couple of days, and the patient is taking food and fluids by mouth, fludrocortisone 0.1 mg/day can be commenced.

Glucose supplementation

Occasionally required because of risk of hypoglycaemia (low glycogen stores in the liver as a result of glucocorticoid deficiency).

Investigate and treat precipitant

This is often infection.

Monitoring treatment

Electrolytes, glucose, and urea.

- Differentiation of secondary from primary adrenal failure can be made more reliably following 3 days i/m ACTH 1 mg. This is because the test relies on the ability of the atrophic adrenal glands to respond to ACTH in secondary adrenocortical failure, whereas in primary adrenal failure, the diseased gland is already maximally stimulated by elevated endogenous levels of ACTH and therefore unable to respond to further stimulation.

- Serum cortisol responses within the first 60 min are superimposable with the short synacthen test.

- There is a progressive rise in cortisol secretion in secondary adrenal insufficiency, but little or no response on primary adrenal insufficiency.

Increased plasma renin activity (assessment of mineralocorticoid sufficiency)

This is one of the earliest abnormalities in developing primary adrenal insufficiency.

Thyroid function tests

Reduced thyroid hormone levels and elevated TSH may be due to a direct effect of glucocorticoid deficiency or due to associated autoimmune hypothyroidism. Re-evaluation is therefore required after adrenal insufficiency has been rectified.

Establish cause of adrenal insufficiency

- *Adrenal autoantibodies* (detect antibodies to adrenal cortex, and more recently specific antibodies to 21-hydroxylase, side-chain-cleavage enzyme, and 17-hydroxylase). 21-Hydroxylase antibodies are the major component of adrenal cortex antibodies. Adrenal cortex antibodies are not detectable in non-autoimmune primary adrenal failure.

- *Imaging*
  - Adrenal enlargement with or without calcification may be seen on CT of the abdomen, suggesting tuberculosis, infiltration or metastatic disease. The adrenals are small and atrophic in autoimmune adrenalitis.
  - Percutaneous CT guided adrenal biopsy is occasionally required.

- *Specific tests*, e.g. serological, or microbiological investigations directed at particular infections, very long chain fatty acids (adrenoleucodystrophy)

Acute adrenal insufficiency

Clinical features
* shock
* hypotension (often not responding to measures such as inotropic support)
* abdominal pain (may present as 'acute abdomen')
* unexplained fever
* often precipitated by major stress such as severe bacterial infection, major surgery, unabsorbed glucocorticoid medication due to vomiting
* occasionally occurs due to bilateral adrenal infarction.

Investigation
* As chronic.
* In the acute situation if the diagnosis is suspected, an inappropriately low cortisol (i.e. <600 nmol/L) is often sufficient to make the diagnosis.
* If the diagnosis is suspected, glucocorticoid therapy with dexamethasone will not interfere with subsequent testing.

Investigation of other associated endocrinopathies

Patients with autoimmune adrenal failure should be investigated for thyroid disease, diabetes mellitus, pernicious anaemia gonadal failure, and parathyroid dysfunction.

Treatment

Maintenance therapy

Glucocorticoid replacement

- Hydrocortisone is the treatment of choice for replacement therapy, as it is reliably and predictably absorbed and allows biochemical monitoring of levels.
- It is administered 3xdaily 10 mg on waking, 5 mg at midday, and 5 mg at 6 p.m.
- An alternative is prednisolone 3 mg on waking and 1–2 mg at 6 p.m. This has the disadvantage that levels cannot be biochemically monitored, but its longer half-life may lead to better suppression of ACTH if pigmentation and markedly elevated morning ACTH levels are a problem. Occasionally dexamethasone is required for this purpose.

Mineralocorticoid replacement

Fludrocortisone (9-flurohydrocortisone) is given at a dose of 0.1 mg daily. Occasionally lower (0.05 mg) or higher (0.2 mg) doses are required.

Monitoring of therapy

Clinical

- For signs of glucocorticoid excess e.g increasing weight
- Blood pressure (including postural change)
- Hypertension and oedema suggest excessive mineralocorticoid replacement, whereas postural hypotension and salt craving suggest insufficient treatment.

Biochemical

- Serum electrolytes
- Plasma renin activity (elevated if insufficient fludrocortisone replacement)
- Cortisol day curve to assess adequacy of treatment (see page 122)
- ACTH levels prior to and following morning glucocorticoids replacement if patient develops increasing pigmentation. If elevated or rising with little suppression following glucocorticoid, MRI scan to exclude rare possibility of pituitary hyperplasia or very rarely the development of a corticotroph adenoma.

Intercurrent illness

* Cortisol requirements increase during severe illness or surgery.
* For moderate elective procedures or investigations, e.g. endoscopy or angiography, patients should receive a single dose of 100 mg hydrocortisone before the procedure.
* For major surgery, patients should take 20 mg hydrocortisone orally or 100 mg intramuscularly with the premedication, and receive 100 mg i/m hydrocortisone 6 hourly for the first 3 days, before reverting rapidly to a maintenance dose.
* To cover severe illness, e.g. pneumonia, patients should receive 50–100 mg hydrocortisone 6 hourly until resolution of the illness.

Pregnancy (see p. 520)

The usual glucocorticoid and mineralocorticoid replacement is continued during pregnancy. Severe hyperemesis gravidarum during the first trimester may require temporary parenteral therapy and patients should be warned about this to avoid precipitation of a crisis. During labour, parenteral glucocorticoid therapy is administered (100 mg i/m every 6 h). Fluid replacement with intravenous 0.9% saline may be required

Education of the patient

* Patient education is the key to successful management. Patients must be taught never to miss a dose. They should be encouraged to wear a MedicAlert bracelet or necklace and always to carry a steroid card.
* Every patient should know how to double the dose of glucocorticoid during febrile ilness, and to get medical attention if unable to take the tablets because of vomiting. They should have a vial of 100 mg hydrocortisone with syringe, diluent, and needle for times when parenteral treatment may be required.

Further reading

Oelkers W. Adrenal insufficiency. *New England Journal of Medicine* 1996; 335: 1206–1212.

Chapter 50

Long-term glucocorticoid administration

Both exogenous glucocorticoid administration and endogenous excess glucocorticoids (Cushing's syndrome) lead to a negative feedback effect on the hypothalamo–pituitary axis (HPA), leading to suppression of both CRH and ACTH secretion and atrophy of the zonae fasiculata and reticularis of the adrenal cortex.

Short-term steroids

• Any patient who has received glucocorticoid treatment for <3 weeks is unlikely to have clinically significant adrenal suppression, and if the medical condition allows it, glucocorticoid treatment can be stopped acutely. A major stress within a week of stopping steroids should, however, be covered with glucocorticoids.

• Exceptions to this are patients who have other possible reasons for adrenocortical insufficiency, who have received more than 40 mg prednisolone (or equivalent), where a short course has been prescribed within 1 year of cessation of long-term therapy, or evening doses (increased HPA axis suppression).

Steroid cover

While receiving glucocorticoid treatment and within 1 year of steroid withdrawal, patients should receive standard steroid supplementation at times of stress, e.g. major trauma, surgery and infection (page 319).

Dehydroepiandrosterone

• DHEA is an abundant circulating adrenal androgen, with a production rate of 25–30 mg/day. Its levels undergo a progressive decline with increasing age, and there has been interest in its physiological role.

• Epidemiological data suggest a link between changes in DHEA and age-related changes including an inverse relationship between DHEA and cardiovascular disease, Alzheimer's disease, and malignancy. Although animal studies have suggested potential therapeutic benefit of DHEA therapy, small studies in humans have so far failed to demonstrate convincing benefit apart from short-term improvement in well-being. Recent evidence suggests that DHEA replacement in patients with Addison's disease may have beneficial effects on well-being.

Long-term steroids

• When patients are receiving supraphysiological doses (>7.5 mg prednisolone, or equivalent) of glucocorticoid, dose reduction depends on disease activity.

• Once a daily equivalent of 7.5 mg prednisolone is reached, the rate of reduction should be slower to allow recovery of the HPA axis.

• If concerned about disease resolution, then the rate of reduction of glucocorticoids is determined by the disease process until 7.5 mg equivalent is reached.

• If the disease has resolved, the dose can be rapidly reduced to 7.5 mg prednisolone by a reduction of 2.5 mg every 3–5 days.

• Once the patient is established on 7.5 mg prednisolone, consider changing to hydrocortisone (20 mg in the morning), as this has a shorter half-life and will therefore lead to less prolonged suppression of ACTH.

• Daily hydrocortisone dose should be reduced by 2.5 mg every 1–2 weeks, or as tolerated until a dose of 10 mg is reached. After 2–3 months a 9 a.m. cortisol is checked 24 h after last dose of hydrocortisone. If it is >300 nmol/L, then hydrocortisone can be stopped and a short synacthen test performed. If the 9 a.m. cortisol is <300 nmol/L, then continue hydrocortisone 10 mg for another 2–3 months and repeat the 9 a.m. cortisol. When basal cortisol is >400 nmol/L, we usually stop regular hydrocortisone and administer in emergency only. Once a short synacthen test demonstrates a normal response, it is helpful to perform an ITT to confirm full recovery of the HPA axis.

Cushing's syndrome

Patients with Cushing's syndrome, whatever the cause, also have HPA axis suppression and may therefore need steroid replacement at times of stress.

Further reading

Baulieu E. DHEA: A fountain of youth? *Journal of Clincal Endocrinology and Metabolism* 1996; 81: 3147–3151.

Nippoldt TB, Nair KS. Is there a case for DHEA replacement? *Ballière's Clinical Endocrinology and Metabolism* 1998; 12: 507–520.

Chapter 51
Adrenal incidentalomas

Definition and epidemiology

- A true incidentaloma, is an incidentally detected lesion with no pathophysiological significance, and needs to be differentiated from incidentally detected but clinically relevant masses.
- The incidental detection of an adrenal mass is becoming more common, as increased numbers of imaging procedures are performed, and with technological improvements in imaging.
- Autopsy studies suggest an incidence of adrenal adenomas of 1–9%.
- Imaging studies suggest an incidence of approximately 3.5%.

Importance

It is important to determine whether the incidentally discovered adrenal mass is

- malignant
- functioning and associated with excess hormonal secretion.

Differential diagnosis of an incidentally detected adrenal nodule

* cortisol-secreting adrenal adenoma causing Cushing's syndrome or subclinical Cushing's syndrome
* CAH
* mineralocorticoid-secreting adrenal adenoma
* androgen-secreting adenoma
* phaeochromocytoma
* adrenal carcinoma
* metastasis
* adrenal cysts
* lipoma
* myelolipoma
* haematoma

Investigation

- Clinical assessment for symptoms and signs of excess hormone secretion and signs of extra-adrenal carcinoma.
- Urinary free cortisol and overnight dexamethasone suppression test, urinary free catecholamines, potassium on 120 mmol sodium day (aldosterone and renin if hypertensive).
- Short synacthen test for 17-hydroxyprogesterone (CAH), and cortisol (for adrenal insufficiency).

Management

- Surgery if evidence of syndrome of hormonal excess attributable to tumour.
- Surgery if diameter of mass >4 cm (increased likelihood of malignancy and definitely if >6 cm in diameter), or imaging features suggestive of malignancy (e.g. lack of clearly circumscribed margin, vascular invasion).
- If size <4 cm, and no sign of excess hormone production, repeat MRI adrenals at 3, 6, 12 and 24 months looking for increase in size.

Chapter 52

Phaeochromocytomas and paragangliomas

Definition

- *Phaeochromocytomas* are adrenomedullary catecholamine-secreting tumours
- *Paragangliomas* are tumours arising from extra-adrenal medullary neural crest derivatives, e.g. organ of Zuckerkandl (sympathetic) or carotid body, aorticopulmonary, intravagal, or jugulotympanic (parasympathetic).

Incidence

Rare tumours, accounting for <0.1% of causes of hypertension. However, it is a very important diagnosis not to be missed as it can be fatal if undiagnosed.

Epidemiology

- Equal sex distribution, and most commonly present in the 3rd and 4th decades. Up to 50% may be diagnosed post-mortem.
- Although the majority (90%) are sporadic, 10% are inherited (Table 52.1).

Table 52.1 Syndromes associated with phaeochromocytomas

Familial phaeochromocytomas	Isolated autosomal dominant trait
MEN-IIa and b p. 731	Mutation in RET proto-oncogene (chromosome 10)
	Hyperparathyroidism and medullary thyroid carcinoma associated with phaeochromocytoma
	MEN IIb also associated with marfanoid phenotype (p. 1132)
Von Hippel–Lindau syndrome p. 711	Mutation of VHL tumour suppressor gene (chromosome 3)
	Renal cell carcinoma, cerebellar haemangioblastoma, retinal angioma, renal and pancreatic cysts
	Phaeochromocytomas in 25%
Neurofibromatosis p. 707	Autosomal dominant condition caused by mutations of NF1 gene on chromosome 17
	Phaechromocytomas in 0.5–1.0%

Pathophysiology

Sporadic tumours are usually unilateral, and <10 cm in diameter. Tumours associated with familial syndromes are more likely to be bilateral, and associated with pre-existing medullary hyperplasia.

Malignancy

* Approximately 15–20% are malignant (less in familial syndromes) and these are characterized by local invasion or distant metastsis rather than capsular invasion. Chromosomal ploidy has been suggested as useful in differentiating benign and malignant tumours.

* Paragangliomas are more likely to be malignant, and to recur.

* Typical sites for metastases are retroperitoneum, lymph nodes, bone, liver, and mediastinum.

Secretory products

* Catecholamine secretion is usually adrenaline or noradrenaline and may be constant or episodic.

* Phenylethanolamine-*N*-methyl transferase (PNMT) is necessary for methylation of noradrenaline to adrenaline, and is cortisol dependent. Small adrenal tumours tend to produce more adrenaline, whereas larger adrenal tumours produce more noradrenaline as a proportion of their blood supply is direct rather than corticomedullary, and therefore lower in cortisol concentrations.

* Paragangliomas (exception – organ of Zuckerkandl) secerete noradrenaline only, as they lack PNMT.

* Pure dopamine secretion is rare, and may be associated with hypotension.

* Other non-catecholamine secretory products may also be produced, including VIP, neuropeptide Y, ACTH (associated with Cushing's syndrome), PTH, and PTHrP.

Clinical features

- Sustained or episodic *hypertension* often resistant to conventional therapy.
- *General*
  - sweating and heat intolerance >80%
  - pallor or flushing
  - feeling of apprehension
  - pyrexia.
- *Neurological* headache (throbbing or constant) (65%), paraesthesiae, visual disturbance, seizures.
- *Cardiovascular* palpitations (65%), chest pain, dyspnoea, postural hypotension.
- *Gastrointestinal* abdominal pain, constipation, nausea.

Complications

- *Cardiovascular* left ventricular failure, dilated cardiomyopathy (reversible), dysrhythmias.
- *Respiratory* pulmonary oedema.
- *Metabolic* carbohydrate intolerance, hypercalcaemia.
- *Neurological* cerebrovascular, hypertensive encephalopathy.

Who should be screened for the presence of a phaeochromocytoma?

+ patients with a family history of MEN, VHL, neurofibromatosis
+ patients with paroxysmal symptoms
+ young patients with hypertension
+ patient developing hypertensive crisis during general anaesthesia/surgery
+ patients with unexplained heart failure.

Factors precipitating a crisis

+ straining
+ exercise
+ pressure on abdomen – tumour palpation, bending over
+ surgery
+ drugs
  – anaesthetics
  – unopposed β-blockade
  – intravenous contrast agents
  – opiates
  – tricyclic antidepressants
  – phenothiazines
  – metoclopramide
  – glucagon

Investigations

Demonstrate catecholamine hypersecretion

24 h urine collection for catecholamines (see opposite)

- Urine is collected into bottles containing acid (warn patient).
- Because of the episodic nature of catecholamine secretion, at least two 24 h collections should be performed. It is useful to perform a collection while a patient is having symptoms, if episodic secretion is suspected.
- The sensitivity of urinary metanephrines and VMAs is less than free catecholamines, and also influenced by dietary intake.
- NB Tricyclic antidepressants and labetalol intefere with adrenaline measurements and should be stopped for 4 days.

Plasma catecholamine measurement

- Intermittent secretion, and the short half-life of catecholamines, makes this test of limited use in screening.
- It can be helpful if drawn while a patient is having a crisis, as normal levels in these circumstances are against the diagnosis. In patients with overt symptoms and signs, plasma catecholamines are usually >2000 pg/mL. However, patients with overt clinical features and plasma catecholamines <1000 pg/mL are unlikely to have a phaeochromocytoma.
- Routine measurement requires controlled conditions – supine and cannulated for 30 min, 10 mL blood drawn into a lithium heparin tube and cold spun.
- NB Plasma catecholamines are elevated by caffeine, nicotine, exercise, and some drugs.

Suppression tests (p. 341)

These tests are useful to differentiate patients who have borderline catecholamine levels.

- *Pentolinium 2.5 mg i/v* Elevated plasma catecholamines at 10 min are seen in phaeochromocytomas, whereas the normal response is suppression into the normal range.
- *Clonidine 300 µg orally* Failure of suppression of plasma catecholamines into the normal range at 120 and 180 min is suggestive of a tumour.

Table 52.2 Substances interfering with urinary catecholamine levels

Increased catecholamines	Decreased catecholamines	Variable effect
α-Blockers	Mono-amine oxidase inhibitors	Levodopa
β-Blockers	Clonidine	Tricyclic antidepressants
Levodopa	Guanethidine and other adrenergic neurone blockers	Phenothiazines
Drugs containing catecholamines, e.g. decongestants		Calcium channel inhibitors
Metoclopramide		ACE inhibitors
Domperidone		Bromocriptine
Hydralazine		
Diazocide		
Nitroglycerine		
Sodium nitroprusside		
Nicotine		
Theophylline		
Caffeine		
Amphetamine		

Table 52.3 Sensitivity and specificity of tests

Test	Sensitivity	Specificity
2 × 24 h urinary free catecholamines	100%	95%
Urinary metanephrines	80%	86%
Urinary VMA	65%	88%
Clonidine suppression test	97%	
MRI	98%	70%
CT	93%	70%
MIBG	80%	95%

Provocative tests (p. 341)

- These are not used routinely as they do not enhance diagnostic accuracy and are potentially dangerous. They should therefore be performed in a specialist unit, under carefully controlled conditions, and covered with calcium channel antagonists.

- Occasionally it may be helpful to perform a glucagon provocation test when negative testing has been associated with high levels of suspicion for the presence of a tumour. A positive glucagon test requires an ×2.5 increase in catecholamines. It is most safely performed with prior α- and β-blockade.

Localization of tumour

Imaging

- These are large tumours, in contrast to Conn's syndrome, and not easily missed with good quality imaging to the bifurcation of the aorta. Approximately 90% will be detected in the abdomen.
- Adrenal imaging should be performed initially, then body imaging (ideally MRI) if tumour not localized in adrenal.
- *MRI* bright hyperintense image on T2.
- *CT* less sensitive and specific – less good at distinguishing between different types of adrenal tumours

^{123}I-MIBG scan

- *meta*-Iodobenzylguanidine is a chromaffin-seeking analogue. Imaging using MIBG is positive in 60–80% phaeochromocytomas, and may locate tumours not visualized on MRI – e.g. multiple and extra-adrenal tumours.
- Performed preoperatively to exclude multiple tumours
- NB Phenoxybenzamine may lead to false negative MIBG imaging, so these scans should be preformed before commencing this drug.

Venous sampling

- Used to localize a phaeochromocytoma/paraganglioma if imaging is unhelpful.
- Caution: α- and β-blockade should be administered before the procedure.
- Reversal of the ratio of noradrenaline : adrenaline ratio (N <1) in the adrenal vein is suggestive of a phaeochromocytoma.

Screening for associated conditions

Up to 23% patients with apparently sporadic phaeochromocytomas may have familial disorders and all patients should therefore be screened for the presence of associated conditons, even if asymptomatic.

MEN

* serum calcium
* serum calcitonin (phaeochromocytomas precede medullary thyroid carcinoma in 10%).

VHL

* opthalmoscopy (retinal angiomas are usually the first manifestation)
* MRI posterior fossa
* ultrasound of kidneys (if not adequately imaged on MRI of adrenals).

Management

Medical

- It is essential that any patient is fully prepared with α- and β-blockade before receiving intravenous contrast, or undergoing a procedure such as venous sampling, or surgery.

- α-Blockade must be commenced before β-blockade to avoid precipitating a hypertensive crisis due to unopposed α-adrenergic stimulation.

- *α-Blockade* commence phenoxybenzamine, as soon as diagnosis made. Start at 10 mg 2× day by mouth, and increase up to 20 mg 4× day.

- *β-Blockade* Commence propanolol 40 mg 8 hourly by mouth 48–72 h after starting phenoxybenzamine.

- Treatment is commenced in hospital. Monitor blood pressure, pulse, and haematocrit. Reversal of α-mediated vasoconstriction may lead to haemodilution. (Check Hb preoperatively).

- To ensure complete blockade before surgery, intravenous *phenoxybenzamine* (0.5 mg/kg over 4 h in 100 mL 5% dextrose) is administered on the 3 days before surgery. There is less experience with competetive α-adrenergic blockade such as prazosin.

Surgical

- Surgical resection is curative in the majority of patients, leading to normotension in at least 75%.

- Mortality from elective surgery is <2%.

- Surgery may be open adrenalectomy, or laparoscopic if the tumour is small and apparently benign. Careful perioperative anaesthetic management is essential as tumour handling may lead to major changes in blood pressure and also occasionally cardiac arrythmias. *Phentolamine* or *nitroprusside* is useful to treat perioperative hypertension, and *esmolol* or *propanolol* for perioperative arrythmias. Hypotension (e.g. after tumour devascularization) usually responds to volume replacement, but occasionally requires inotropic support.

Follow-up

- Cure is assessed by 24 h urine free catecholamine measurement, but since catecholamines may remain elevated for up to 10 days follow-

Test procedures

Clonidine suppression test

* patient supine and cannulated for 30 min
* clonidine 300 μg orally
* plasma catecholamines measured at time 0, 120, and 180 min
* failure to suppress into the normal range is suggestive of a tumour
* 1.5% false positive rate in patients with essential hypertension

Pentolinium suppression test

* patient supine and cannulated for 30 min
* pentolinium 2.5 mg i/v
* plasma catecholamines measured at time 0 and 10 min
* failure to suppress into the normal range is suggestive of a tumour

Glucagon provocation test

* caution – may provoke a crisis
* patients should have received full α- and β-blockade before the test is performed
* patient supine and canulated for 30 min
* glucagon 1 mg i/v at time 0
* plasma catecholamines measured at 0, 2, 4, 6, 8, and 10 min
* catecholamine levels rise in patients with phaeochromo-cyotomas

ing surgery, these should not be performed until 2 weeks post-operatively.

• Lifelong follow-up is essential to detect recurrence of a benign tumour, or metastasis from a malignant tumour, as it is impossible to exclude malignancy on a histological specimen.

Malignancy

• Malignant tumours require long-term α- and β-blockade. The tyrosine kinase inhibitor α-*methylparatyrosine* may help control symptoms.

• High dose ^{131}I MIBG can be used to treat metastatic disease, although results can be disappointing.

• Chemotherapy using *cyclophosphamide, vincristine, adriamycin*, and *dacarbazine* has been associated with symptomatic improvement.

• Radiotherapy can be useful palliation in patients with bony metastases.

Prognosis

• Hypertension may persist in 25% patients who have undergone successful tumour removal.

• 5 year survival for 'benign' tumours is 96%, and the recurrence rate is <10%.

• 5 year survival for malignant tumours is 44%.

Further reading

Bouloux PMG, Fakeeh M. Investigation of phaeochormocytoma. *Clinical Endocrinology* 1995; 43: 657–664.

Neumann HPH, Berger DP, Sigmund G, Blum U, Schmidt D, Parmer RJ, Volk B, Kirste G. Phaeochromocytomas, multiple endocrine neoplasia type 2 and Von Hippel–Lindau disease *New England Journal of Medicine* 1993; 329: 1531–1538.

Young WF. Phaeochromocytoma and primary aldosteronism: diagnostic approaches. *Endocrinology and Metabolism Clinics of North America* 1997; 26: 801–827.

Part IV
Reproductive endocrinology

Chapter 53
Hirsutism

Definition

Hirsutism (not a diagnosis in itself) is the presence of excess hair growth in women as a result of increased androgen production and increased skin sensitivity to androgens.

Physiology of hair growth

Before puberty the body is covered by fine unpigmented hairs, or vellus hairs. These, in addition to eyebrows and eyelashes, are not dependent on androgens for growth. During adolescence, androgens convert vellus hairs into coarse, pigmented terminal hairs in androgen-dependent areas. The extent of terminal hair growth depends on the concentration and duration of androgen exposure as well as on the sensitivity of the individual hair follicle. The reason different body regions respond differently to the same androgen concentration is unknown but may be related to the number of androgen receptors in the hair follicle. Genetic factors play an important role in the individual susceptibility to circulating androgens, as evidenced by racial differences in hair growth.

Androgen production in women

In females, testosterone is secreted primarily by the ovaries and adrenal glands although a significant amount is produced by the peripheral conversion of androstenedione and dehydroepiandrostenedione (DHEA). Ovarian androgen production is regulated by luteneizing hormone, whereas adrenal production is ACTH dependent. The predominant androgens produced by the ovaries are testosterone and androstenedione, and the adrenal glands are the main source of dehydroepiandrostenedione. Circulating testosterone is mainly bound to sex hormone binding globulin (SHBG) and it is the free testosterone which is biologically active. To be active, testosterone is converted to the more potent dihydrotestosterone in the skin by the enzyme 5α-reductase. Androstenedione and DHEA are not significantly protein-bound.

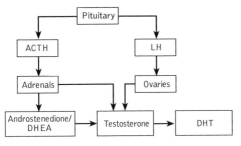

Fig. 53.1 Regulation of andogen production in women.

Signs of virilization

* frontal balding
* deepening of voice
* increased muscle size
* clitoromegaly

Causes of androgen-independent hair growth

* drugs, e.g. phenytoin, cyclosporin, glucocorticoids
* anorexia nervosa
* hypothyroidism
* familial

Table 53.1 Causes of hirsutism

Ovarian	Polycystic ovary syndrome	95%
	Androgen-secreting tumours	<1%
Adrenal	Congenital adrenal hyperplasia	<1%
	Cushing's syndrome	<1%
	Androgen-secreting tumours	<1%
	Acromegaly	1%

Evaluation

Androgen-dependent hirsutism

Normally develops following puberty. Hairs are coarse and pigmented and typically grow in areas where men develop hair growth. It is often accompanied by other evidence of androgen excess such as acne, oily skin and male pattern alopecia.

Androgen-independent hair growth

Excess vellus hairs over face and trunk including forehead. It does not respond to anti-androgen treatment.

History

• *Age and rate of onset of hirsutism* Slowly progressive hirsutism following puberty suggests a benign cause, whereas rapidly progressive hirsutism of recent onset requires further immediate investigation to rule out an androgen-secreting neoplasm.

• *Menstrual history* ?oligomenorrhoeic.

• Presence of other evidence of *hyperandrogenism*, e.g. acne or bitemporal alopecia.

• *Drug history* Some progestins used in oral contraceptive preparations may be androgenic (e.g. norethisterone).

Physical examination

• Distinguish beween *androgen-dependent* and *androgen-independent* hair growth.

• Assess the *extent and severity* of hirsutism. The Ferriman–Gallwey score (see table) assesses the degree of hair growth in 11 regions of the body. This provides a semi-objective method of monitoring disease progression and treatment outcome.

• *Virilization* should be looked for, as this indicates severe hyperandrogenism and should be further investigated.

• *Acanthosis nigricans* is indicative of insulin resistance and probable polycystic ovary syndrome.

• *Rare causes* of hyperandrogenism such as Cushing's syndrome and acromegaly should be ruled out.

Table 53.2 Assessment of hirsutism (from Ferriman-Gallwey, 1961)

Site	Grade	Definition
Upper lip	1	A few hairs at outer margin
	2	A small moustache at outer margin
	3	A moustache extending halfway from outer margin
	4	A moustache extending to midline
Chin	1	A few scattered hairs
	2	Scattered hairs with small concentrations
	3	Complete cover, light
	4	Complete cover, heavy
Chest	1	Circumareolar hairs
	2	With midline hair
	3	Fusion of these areas
	4	Complete cover
Upper back	1	A few scattered hairs
	2	More, but still scattered
	3	Complete cover, light
	4	Complete cover, heavy
Lower back	1	Sacral tuft of hair
	2	Some lateral extension
	3	Three-quarter cover
	4	Complete cover
Upper abdomen	1	A few midline hairs
	2	Rather more, still midline
	3	Half cover
	4	Full cover
Lower abdomen	1	A few midline hairs
	2	A midline streak of hair
	3	A midline band of hair
	4	An inverted V-shaped growth
Arm	1	Sparse growth affecting not more than a quarter of the limb surface
	2	More than this, cover still incomplete
	3	Complete cover, light
	4	Complete cover, heavy
Forearm	1,2,3,4	Complete cover of dorsal surface, 2 grades of light and 2 grades of heavy growth
Thigh	1,2,3,4	As for arm
Leg	1,2,3,4	As for arm
Total score		

Laboratory investigation

Serum testosterone should be measured in all women. If this is <5 nmol/L then the risk of a sinister cause for her hirsutism is minimal. Further investigations and management of the individual disorders will be discussed in the following chapters.

Further reading

Ferriman DG, *Journal of Clinical Endocrinology and Metabolism* 1961; 21(11): 1440–1447.

Chapter 54
Polycystic ovary syndrome

Definition

- A heterogenous clinical syndrome characterized by hyperandrogenism and ovulatory dysfunction in which other causes of androgen excess have been excluded.
- The diagnosis is further supported by the presence of characteristic ovarian morphology on ultrasound.

Epidemiology

PCOS is the most common endocrinopathy in women of reproductive age. 95% of women presenting to outpatients with hirsutism have polycystic ovary syndrome. The estimated prevalence of PCOS ranges from 8% on clinical criteria alone, to 22% on ultrasonic diagnosis.

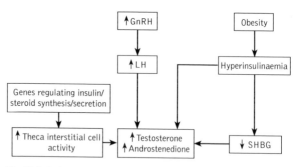

Fig. 54.1 Pathogenesis of PCOS.

Pathogenesis

Genetic

• PCOS is an oligogenic or polygenic disorder.

• Insulin synthesis genes and steroid enzyme biosynthesis gene are likely candidates, e.g. *INS*, *VNTR*, and *CYP11* genes.

Hyperandrogenism

• The main source of hyperandrogenaemia is the ovaries although there may also be adrenal androgen hypersecretion.

• The biochemical basis of ovarian dysfunction is unclear. Studies suggest an abnormality of cytochrome P-450c17α activity but this is unlikely to be the primary event but rather an index of increased steroidogenesis by ovarian theca cells.

• There is also an increase in the frequency and amplitude of GnRH pulses, resulting in the increase in LH concentration which is characteristic of the syndrome. This is probably secondary to anovulation and low progesterone levels.

Hyperinsulinaemia

• Insulin and IGF-1 receptors are found in abundance in the ovarian stroma and it has been shown that insulin, in the presence of LH, stimulates ovarian production of androgens. This is exaggerated in PCOS.

• Insulin also diminishes SHBG levels with a consequent rise in free androgen levels.

Features

- *Onset of symptoms* Symptoms often begin around puberty, after weight gain or after stopping the oral contraceptive pill but can present at any time.

- *Oligo/amenorrhoea* (70%) Due to anovulation. These women are well-oestrogenized so there is no risk of osteoporosis, unlike other causes of amenorrhoea.

- *Hirsutism* (60%)
  - 25% of women also suffer from acne or male pattern alopecia. Virilization is not a feature of PCOS.
  - There is often a family history of hirsutism or irregular periods. Hirsutism secondary to adrenal or ovarian tumours is usually rapidly progressive, associated with virilization and higher testosterone concentrations.
  - 1% of hirsute women have non-classical congenital adrenal hyperplasia(see p. 366) and this should be excluded particularly in women with significantly raised serum testosterone levels.

- *Obesity* (35%) Symptoms worsen with obesity as it is accompanied by increased testosterone concentrations as a result of the associated hyperinsulinaemia.

- *Infertility* (30%) Due to anovulation.

Rule out an androgen-secreting tumour

If there is:

* evidence of virilization
* testosterone >5 nmol/L (or >3 nmol/L in postmenopausal women)
* rapidly progressive hirsutism
* *MRI of adrenals and ovaries* will detect adrenal or ovarian tumours >1 cm.
* *Selective venous sampling:*
    - Occasionally necessary to locate virilizing tumours undetected by imaging.
    - Blood samples are taken from both adrenal and ovarian veins and from the peripheral circulation.
    - A virilizing tumour is likely if an androgen concentration gradient is detected

Table 54.1 Pharmacological treatment of hirsutism

Ovarian androgen suppression	Oral contraceptive pill
	GnRH analogues
Adrenal androgen suppression	Glucocorticoids
Androgen receptor blockers	Cyproterone acetate
	Spironolactone
	Flutamide
5α-reductase inhibitors	Finasteride

Investigations

The aims of investigations are threefold: to confirm the diagnosis, to exclude serious underlying disorders, and to screen for complications.

Confirmation of diagnosis

* *Testosterone concentration*
  - Performed primarily as a screen for the presence of other causes of hyperandrogenism.
  - Women with PCOS may have normal serum testosterone levels and serum androgen concentrations do not necessarily reflect the degree of hirsutism.
* *LH concentration*
  - Raised in 50–70% of anovulatory patients with reversal of the FSH/LH ratio.
  - The higher the LH level the more likely the risk of anovulation and infertility. Cannot be used alone to diagnose PCOS since it is normal in half the patients.
* *SHBG*
  - Low in 50% of women with PCOS owing to the hyperinsulinaemic state, with a consequent increase in circulating free androgens.
* *Pelvic ultrasound of ovaries and endometrium*
  - 91% sensitivity in experienced hands, with transvaginal ultrasounds giving the highest yield.
  - Ultrasonic diagnosis of PCOS is made by the presence of >8 follicular cysts of <10 mm and increased ovarian stroma.
  - Measurement of endometrial thickness is also useful in the diagnosis of endometrial hyperplasia in the presence of anovulation. Endometrial hyperplasia is diagnosed if the endometrial thickness is >10 mm.
  - Transvaginal ultrasound will also identify 90% of ovarian virilizing tumours.

Exclusion of serious underlying disease

* *Serum prolactin*
  - In the presence of infertility or oligoamenorrhoea.
  - Mild hyperprolactinaemia (up to 2000 mU/L) is present in up to 30% of women with PCOS, and dopamine agonist treatment of this may be necessary if pregnancy is desired.

- *17 OH (17OHP) progesterone level*
  - Used to exclude late onset congenital adrenal hyperplasia.
  - Indicated in those with testosterone concentrations in excess of 5 nmol/L or with evidence of virilization.
  - May also perform a synacthen test looking for an exaggerated rise in 17 OHP in response to ACTH in the presence of non-classic 21-hydroxylase deficiency (see p. 366).
  - If the patient is ovulating then all 17OHP measurements should be performed during the follicular phase of the cycle to avoid false positives.

- *DHEAS and androstenedione concentrations*
  - Both can be moderately raised in PCOS. DHEAS is a useful adrenal marker of hyperandrogenism. In cases of suspected tumours levels are usually in excess of 20 μmol/L.

- *Other*
  - Depending on clinical suspicion, e.g urinary free cortisol or overnight dexamethasone suppression test if Cushing's syndrome is suspected, but not routinely.

Screening for complications

- *Serum lipids and blood glucose*
  - Insulin resistance increases the risk of type 2 diabetes mellitus and hypertriglyceridaemia.
  - Up to 40% of women with PCOS have impaired glucose tolerance and up to 10% have frank diabetes mellitus.

Management

Weight loss

Weight loss in obese patients will reduce insulin resistance and thus hyperandrogenaemia. Obese women are less likely to respond to antiandrogens and infertility treatment. With a loss of 5% of their starting weight, women with PCOS show a 40% improvement in their hirsutism. Restoration of menstrual regularity and fertility can be acheived by weight loss alone.

Insulin sensitizers

In obese and lean women with PCOS and insulin resistance, metformin (500 mg 3x daily) may improve insulin sensitivity with a corresponding reduction in serum androgen and LH concentrations and an increase in SHBG levels. It may also regulate menstruation by improving ovulatory function and thus inducing fertility. No long-term studies have been done on its effect on hirsutism. Its effects seem to be independent of weight reduction, although the benefits are greatest when weight reduction occurs in obese women. However, there have been very few controlled trials using metformin in PCOS and all trials have been limited by small numbers of subjects. Women should be warned of its gastrointestinal side-effects. In order to minimize these, they should be started on a low dose (500 mg once daily) which may be increased gradually to a therapeutic dose over a number of weeks.

Troglitazone is a thiazolidinedione, another insulin sensitizer which has shown encouraging effects on menstruation and fertility in women with PCOS. However, it has been withdrawn from both the UK and US markets because of liver problems. Other thiazolidinediones may in the future be used in the treatment of PCOS.

Hirsutism

Pharmacological treatment of hirsutism is directed at slowing the growth of new hair but has little impact on established hair. It should be combined with mechanical methods of hair removal such as electrolysis and laser therapy. Therapy is most effective when started early. There is slow improvement over the first 6–12 months of treatment. Patients should be warned that facial hair is slow to respond, treatment is prolonged, and symptoms may recur after discontinuation of drugs. Adequate contraception is mandatory during pharmacological treatment of hirsutism because of possible teratogenicity.

Ovarian androgen suppression

- *Oral contraceptive pill (OCP)*
  - The oestrogen component increases SHBG levels and thus reduces free androgen concentrations; the progestogen component inhibits LH secretion and thus ovarian androgen production.
  - Dianette, which contains cyproterone acetate (2 mg), is preferred.
  - The effect of the OCP alone on hair growth is modest at best, so it may be combined with an antiandrogen (see below). Avoid OCP with androgenic progestagen.

- *GnRH analogues*
  - Suppress gonadotrophin secretion and thus ovarian androgen production.
  - Rarely used. They cause oestrogen deficiency so have to be combined with 'add-back' oestrogen treatment. Also, they are expensive and need to be given parenterally.
  - Use is confined to women with severe hyperandrogenism in whom antiandrogens have been ineffective or not tolerated.

Adrenal androgen suppression

- *Glucocorticoids* Suppress adrenal androgen production. However, the effect on hirsutism is minimal and there is the risk of hypothalamic-pituitary-adrenal suppression. Steroids may worsen hyperinsulinaemia, thus exacerbating ovarian androgen excess.

Androgen receptor blockers

These are most effective when combined with oral contraceptives. All are contraindicated in pregnancy. They act by competitively inhibiting the binding of testosterone and dihydrotestosterone to the androgen receptor.

- *Cyproterone acetate (CPA)*
  - A progestagen which also increases *hepatic androgen clearance*.
  - *Dose* 25–100 mg for last 10 days of the menstrual cycle in combination with the OCP.
  - *Side-effects* Amenorrhoea if given alone for prolonged periods or in higher doses. *Progesterone side-effects* Hepatic toxicity rare, but monitoring of liver function 6 monthly is recommended.
  - A *washout period* of 3–4 months is recommended prior to attempting conception.

- *Spironolactone*
  - weak antiandrogen
  - *Dose* 50–200 mg a day.

- *Side-effects* polymenorrhoea if not combined with the OCP. A fifth of women complain of GI symptoms when on high doses of spironolactone. Potassium levels should be monitored and other potassium-sparing drugs should be avoided.

* *Flutamide*
  - A potent antiandrogen.
  - *Dose* 125 mg a day.
  - *Side-effects* Dry skin, nausea in 10%. However, there is a 0.4% risk of hepatic toxicity and it should therefore be used with extreme caution.

5α-reductase inhibitors

Block the conversion of testosterone to the more potent androgen, dihydrotestosterone.

* *Finasteride*
  - *Dose* 5 mg a day. Is at least as effective as CPA.
  - *Side-effects* no significant adverse effects.
  - Can be used as monotherapy and is therefore of value if the OCP is contraindicated. However, adequate contraceptive measures are mandatory because of its teratogenicity. In addition, pregnancy should not be attempted until at least 3 months after drug cessation.
  - Further experience is required before recommending it as first line therapy.

Amenorrhoea

* Associated with endometrial hyperplasia.
* Threefold increased risk of endometrial carcinoma.
* A minimum of a withdrawal bleed every 3 months minimizes the risk of endometrial neoplasia
* *Treatment*
  - OCP
  - Metformin (500 mg 3× daily)
  - *Alternatives* A progestogen may be added for the latter half of the cycle. However, there is the risk of exacerbating hirsutism. Less androgenic progestogens include *dydrogesterone* (Duphaston) and *medroxyprogesterone e.g.* Medroxyprogesterone 20 mg last 14/7 of 3 mth cycle (Provera). Norethisterone should be avoided.

Infertility

Ovulation induction regimens are indicated. Obesity adversely affects fertility outcome with poorer pregnancy rates and higher rates of spontaneous abortions so weight reduction should be strongly encouraged.

- *Clomiphene citrate*
  - Inhibits oestrogen negative feedback, increasing FSH secretion and thus stimulating ovarian follicular growth.
  - *Dose* 25–150 mg a day from day 5 of menstrual cycle for 5 days.
  - *Response rates* 80% of women with PCOS will ovulate, although the pregnancy rate is only 67%. Recent studies have shown that treatment with metformin may improve response to clomphene in resistant cases.
  - *Complications* Risk of ovarian neoplasia following prolonged clomiphene treatment remains unclear, so limit treatment to a maximum of 6 cycles.

- *Gonadotrophin preparations (hMG or FSH)*
  - Used in those unresponsive to clomiphene. Low dose regimes show better response rates and less complications., e.g. 75 IU/day for 2 weeks then increase by 37.5 IU/day every 7 days as required.
  - 94% ovulation rate and 40% conception rate after 4 cycles.
  - *Complications* hyperstimulation, multiple pregnancies.
  - Close ultrasonic monitoring is essential.

- *Surgery*
  - Laparoscopic ovarian diathermy or laser drilling may restore ovulation in up to 90% of women with cumulative pregnancy rates of 80% within 8 months of treatment.
  - *Complications* surgical adhesions, although usually mild.

- *In vitro fertilization*
  - In the minority of women who fail to respond to ovulation induction.
  - 60–80% conception rate after 6 cycles.

Prognosis and follow up

- The natural history of untreated hirsutism is that of a gradual progression up until the time of the menopause, following which there is gradual improvement apart from facial hair, which continues to progress.
- Follow-up studies of postmenopausal women with histological evidence of PCOS show a 15% prevalence of type 2 diabetes mellitus, compared with <2% in the general population. These studies also revealed a significantly increased prevalence of hypertension in

women with PCOS. It therefore seems prudent to monitor blood pressure on a regular basis and have a baseline fasting blood glucose and serum lipid profile.

• Long term follow-up of women with PCOS has revealed that they are apparently not at increased risk of developing ischaemic heart disease despite the presence of multiple risk factors.

Further reading

Barnes RB. Diagnosis and therapy of hyperandrogenism. *Baillière's Clinical Obstetric Gynaecology* 1997; 11(2): 369–396.

Conn JJ, Jacobs HS. The clinical management of hirsutism. *European Journal of Endocrinology* 1997; 136: 339–348.

Dahlgren E, Johansson S, Lindstedt G *et al.* Women with polycystic ovary syndrome wedge resected in 1956 to 1965: a long term follow up focusing on natural history and circulating hormones. *Fertility and Sterility* 1992; 57(3): 505–513.

Dunaif A. Insulin resistance and polycystic ovary syndrome: mechanism and implications for pathogenesis. *Endocrine Review* 1997; 18(6): 774–800.

Ehrmann DA. Insulin lowering therapeutic modalities for polycystic ovary syndrome. *Endocrinology and Metabolism Clinics of North America* 1999; 28(2):423–438.

Franks S, Gharani N, Waterworth D *et al.* The genetic basis of polycystic ovary syndrome. *Human Reproduction* 1997; 12(12): 2641–2648.

Pierpoint T, McKeigue PM, Isaacs AJ, Wild SH, Jacobs HS. Mortality of women with polycystic ovary syndrome at long term follow up. *Journal of Clinical Epidemiology* 1998; 51(7): 581–586.

Chapter 55
Congenital adrenal hyperplasia in adults

Definition

CAH is an inherited group of disorders characterized by a deficiency of one of the enzymes necessary for cortisol biosynthesis.

* >90% of cases are due to 21α-hydroxylase deficiency.
* Wide clinical spectrum, from presentation in neonatal period with salt wasting and virilization to non-classic CAH in adulthood.
* Inherited in an autosomal recessive manner.

Epidemiology

* Wide racial variations, most common in those of Jewish origin.
* Carrier frequency of classic CAH 1 : 60 in white people.
* Carrier frequency of non-classic CAH 19% in Ashkenazi Jews, 13.5% in Hispanics, 6% in Italians and 3% in other white people.

Pathogenesis

Genetics

* *CYP21* encodes for the 21α-hydroxylase enzyme, located on the short arm of chromosome 6 (chromosome 6p21.3). In close proximity is the *CYP21* pseudogene, with 90% homology but no functional activity.
* 21α-hydroxylase deficiency results from gene mutations, partial gene deletions or gene conversions in which sequences from the pseudogene are transferred to the active gene, rendering it inactive. There is a correlation between the severity of the molecular defect and the clinical severity of the disorder. Non-classic CAH is usually due to a point mutation (single base change) whereas a gene conversion or partial deletion usually results in presentation in infancy with salt wasting or severe virilization.

Biochemistry

See Fig. 55.1.

21α-hydroxylase deficiency results in aldosterone and cortisol deficiency. There is ACTH oversecretion because of the loss of negative feedback, and this causes adrenocortical hyperplasia and excessive accumulation of 17-hydroxy progesterone (17OHP) and other steroid precursors. These are then shunted into androgen synthesis pathways resulting in testosterone and androstenedione excess.

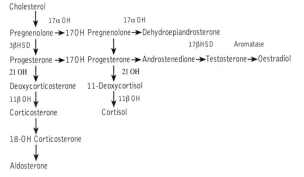

Fig 55.1 Adrenal steroid biosynthesis pathway. 3βHSD, 3β-hydroxysteroid dehydrogenase; 21 OH, 21-hydroxylase; 11β OH, 11β-hydroxylase; 17α OH, 17α-hydroxylase; 17β HSD, 17β-hydroxysteroid dehydrogenase.

Clinical presentation

Classic CAH

* Most patients are diagnosed in infancy, and their clinical presentation is discussed elsewhere (see p. 654).

* *Problems persisting into adulthood* sexual dysfunction and subfertility in females, particularly in salt wasters. Reconstructive genital surgery is required in the majority of women who were virilized at birth to create an adequate vaginal introitus. With improvement of medical and surgical care, pregnancy rates have improved. Fertility rates of 60% have been reported in women with classic CAH.

* In males, high levels of adrenal androgens suppress gonadotrophins and thus testicular function. Spermatogenesis may therefore be affected if CAH is poorly controlled.

Non-classic CAH

* Due to partial deficiency of 21α-hydroxylase.

* Present with hirsutism (82%), acne (25%), and oligomenorrhoea (50%), often around the onset of puberty. Subfertility due to anovulation occurs in 50% of untreated patients.

* A third of women have polycystic ovaries on ultrasound and adrenal incidentalomas or hyperplasia are seen in 40%.

* *Asymptomatic in males* The effect of non-classic CAH on male fertility is unknown.

Investigations

Because of the diurnal variation in adrenal hormonal secretion, all investigations should be performed at 9 a.m.

Diagnosis of non-classic CAH – 17OHP measurement

Timing of measurement

- Screen in the follicular phase of the menstrual cycle. 17OHP is produced by the corpus luteum, so false positive results may occur if measured in the luteal phase of the cycle.
- Must be measured at 9 a.m. to avoid false negative results as 17OHP has a diurnal variation similar to that of ACTH.

Interpretation of result

<5 nmol/L normal

>15 nmol/L   CAH

5–15 nmol/L   proceed to ACTH stimulation test. A fifth will have non-classic CAH.

ACTH stimulation test

- Measure 17OHP 60 min after ACTH administration.
- An exaggerated rise in 17OHP is seen in non-classic CAH.
- 17OHP level <30 nmol/L post-ACTH excludes the diagnosis.
- Most patients have levels >45 nmol/L.
- Levels of 30–45 nmol/L suggest heterozygosity.
- Cortisol response to ACTH stimulation is usually low-normal.

Other investigations

Androgens

- In poorly controlled classic CAH in women, testosterone and androstenedione levels may be in the adult male range. Dehydroepiandrosterone sulphate levels are usually only mildly, and not consistently, elevated in CAH.
- Circulating testosterone and, particularly androstenedione, are elevated in non-classic CAH, but there is a large overlap with levels seen in PCOS so serum androgen concentrations cannot be used to distinguish between the disorders.

Renin

* Plasma renin levels are markedly elevated in 75% of patients with inadequately treated classic CAH, reflecting deficient aldosterone production.
* A proportion of women with non-classic CAH may also have mildly elevated renin concentrations.

ACTH

* Greatly elevated in poorly controlled classic CAH.
* Usually normal levels in non-classic CAH.

Table 55.1 Enzyme deficiencies in CAH

Enzyme deficiency	Incidence (per births)	Clinical features
Classic 21α-hydroxylase	1 : 10 000–1 : 15 000	Salt wasting, ambiguous genitalia in females, precocious pubarche in males
Non-classic 21α-hydroxylase (partial deficiency)	1 : 27–1 : 1000	Hirsutism, oligomenorrhoea in pubertal girls, asymptomatic in boys
11ß-hydroxylase	1 : 100 000	Ambiguous genitalia, virilization, hypertension
3ß-hydroxylase	Rare	Mild virilization, salt wasting in severe cases
17α-hydroxylase	Rare	Delayed puberty in females, pseudohermaphroditism in males, hypertension, hypokalaemia

Management

The aims of treatment of CAH in adulthood are:

* to maintain normal energy levels and weight and avoid adrenal crises in all patients
* to minimize hyperandrogenism and to restore regular menses and fertility in women
* to avoid glucocorticoid over-replacement.

Classic CAH

* *Prednisolone*, total dose 5–7.5 mg/day. Given in two divided doses, with a third of the total dose given on waking (about 7 a.m.) and two-thirds of the dose on retiring. The aim is to suppress the early morning peak of ACTH and thus androgen secretion. Occasional patients who are not controlled on prednisolone may be optimally treated with nocturnal dexamethasone instead (0.5 mg).

* As with other forms of adrenal insufficiency, glucocorticoid doses should be doubled during illness. This is discussed in detail elsewhere (p. 319).

* 75% of patients are salt wasters and thus require mineralocorticoid replacement therapy. Fludrocortisone in a dose of 50–200 µg/day is given as a single daily dose. The aim is to keep plasma renin levels in the mid-normal range.

* Bilateral adrenalectomy may very occasionally be considered in patients with severe virilization.

Non-classic CAH

* *Oligo/amenorrhoea* Glucocorticoid therapy, e.g. noctural dexamethasone 0.25–0.5 mg or prednisolone 2.5–5 mg/day, may be used. Slightly higher doses may be required to normalize ovulatory function.

* *Hirsutism and acne* May alternatively, and more effectively, be treated using antiandrogens, e.g. cyproterone acetate combined with oral oestrogens (see management of PCOS, p. 359). Spironolactone should be avoided because of the potential risk of salt wasting and thus hyperreninaemia.

* If plasma renin level is elevated then fludrocortisone given in a dose sufficient to normalize renin concentrations may improve adrenal hyperandrogenism.

* Males do not usually require treatment.

Management of pregnancy in CAH

Indications for prenatal treatment

* *Maternal classic CAH* Screen partner using basal ± ACTH-stimulated 17OHP levels (see investigations above). If levels elevated, proceed to genotyping. If heterozygote, then prenatal treatment of foetus recommended.
* Previous child from same partner with CAH

Aims of prenatal treatment (p. 372)

* Prevention of virilization of an affected female foetus.

Treatment (commenced before 10 weeks gestation)

* Dexamethasone (20 μg/kg) crosses the placenta to reduce foetal adrenal hyperandrogenism.

Outcome

* 50% of affected females do not require reconstructive surgery.

Complications

* No known foetal congenital malformations from dexamethasone treatment.
* Subtle effects of glucocorticoids on neuropsychological function unknown.
* Maternal complications of glucocorticoid excess in 1%, e.g. mood swings and weight gain. Some suggest reducing the dose of dexamethasone in the third trimester of pregnancy in order to reduce the risk of maternal complications. However, the efficacy of this regime in preventing neonatal virilization has not been proven.

There is debate about whether women with non-classic CAH should be offered prenatal treatment with dexamethasone. There have been no cases of women with non-classic CAH giving birth to a virilized female. Additionally, the estimated risk of conceiving an infant with classic CAH is 1 : 1000. As the risk of foetal virilization is therefore low, dexamethasone treatment of this group of women seems unwarranted. However, these infants should be screened in the neonatal period by measuring 17OHP levels.

Monitoring of treatment

Annual follow up is usually adequate in adults.

• *Clinical assessment* Look for evidence of hyperandrogenism and glucocorticoid excess. Amenorrhoea in females usually suggests inadequate therapy.

• *17OHP* Aim for a mildly elevated level (about 2× normal). Normalizing 17OHP will result in complications from supra-physiological doses of glucocorticoids.

• *Plasma renin* Aim for renin in mid-normal range. Hyper-androgenism will be difficult to control if patient is mildly salt-depleted (ACTH production stimulated by hypovolaemia).

• *Androgens* Aim to normalize serum androstenedione taken before a.m. steroids.

Prenatal treatment protocol

Start dexamethasone 20μg/kg per day (prepregnancy weight)
Best results if started at 4–6 weeks, certainly before week 9 of gestation

↓

Chorionic villus sampling at 10–12 weeks for
fetal karyotype
DNA analysis

↓	↓	↓
46XX, unaffected	46XY	46XX, affected (1 in 8)
↓	↓	↓
	Discontinue treatment	Continue treatment to term

Fig 55.2 Prenatal treatment protocol.

Prognosis

Adults with treated CAH have a normal life expectancy. Improvement in medical and surgical care has also improved quality of life for most sufferers. However, there are a few unresolved issues:

* *Height* Despite optimal treatment in childhood, patients with CAH are, on average, significantly shorter than their predicted genetic height. Studies suggest that this may be due to overtreatment with glucocorticoids during infancy.

* *Fertility* Remains reduced in females with CAH, particularly in salt wasters, due to factors including inadequate vaginal introitus and anovulation secondary to both hyperandrogenism and high 17OHP levels. Fertility may also be affected in males with poorly controlled classic CAH.

* *Adrenal incidentalomas and testicular adrenal rest tumours* Benign adrenal adenomas have been reported in up to 50% of patients with classic CAH. Males with classic CAH may develop gonadal adrenocortical rests which may be misdiagnosed as testicular tumours. These are ACTH-responsive and should be treated by optimizing glucocorticoid therapy.

* *Psychosexual issues* There is an increased propensity for gender identity disorders. In animal studies, prenatal exposure of genetic females to testosterone during critical periods of development enhances masculine behaviour. Females with classic CAH also show an increased tendency to male pattern behaviour. A significant number of women with classic CAH, despite adequacy of vaginal reconstruction, are not sexually active.

Further reading

Azziz R, Dewailly D, Owerbach D. Non-classic adrenal hyperplasia: current concepts. *Journal of Clinical Endocrinology and Metabolism* 1994; 78(4): 810–815.

Hunt PJ, Inder WJ. Diagnosis, monitoring and management of congenital adrenal hyperplasia. *Current Opinions in Endocrinology and Diabetes* 1995; 2: 231–238.

Premawaradhana LDKE, Hughes IA, Read GF, Scanlon MF. Longer term outcome in females with congenital adrenal hyperplasia: the Cardiff experience. *Clinical Endocrinology* 1997; 46: 327–332.

Van Wyk JJ, Gunther DF, Ritzen EM, Wedell A, Cutler GB, Migeon CJ. The use of adrenalectomy as treatment for congenital adrenal hyperplasia. *Journal of Clinical Endocrinology and Metabolism* 1996; 81(9): 3180–3190.

Chapter 56
Androgen-secreting tumours

Definition

Rare tumours of the ovary or adrenal gland which may be benign or malignant, which cause virilization in women through androgen production.

Epidemiology and pathology

Androgen secreting ovarian tumours

- 75% develop before the age of 40 years.
- Account for 0.4% of all ovarian tumours. 20% are malignant.
- Tumours are 5–25 cm in size. The larger they are, the more likely they are to be malignant. They are rarely bilateral.
- Two major types:
  - sex cord stromal cell tumours: often contain testicular cell types
  - adrenal-like tumours: often contain adrenocortical or Leydig cells.
- Other tumours, e.g. gonadoblastomas and teratomas, may also on occasion present with virilization.

Androgen secreting adrenal tumours

- 50% develop before the age of 50 years.
- Larger tumours, particularly >6 cm, are more likely to be malignant.

Clinical features

- *Onset of symptoms* Usually recent onset of rapidly progressive symptoms.
- *Hyperandrogenism*
  - hirsutism of varying degree, often severe (Ferriman–Gallwey score) (p. 346); male pattern balding and acne are also common.
  - usually oligo-amenorrhoea
  - infertility may be a presenting feature.
- *Virilization* (p. 347) indicates severe hyperandrogenism is associated with clitoromegaly and is present in 98% of women with androgen-producing tumours. Not usually a feature of PCOS.
- *Other*
  - abdominal pain
  - palpable abdominal mass
  - ascites
  - symptoms and signs of Cushing's syndrome are present in 50% of women with adrenal tumours.

Investigations

See Fig. 56.1 on facing page.

Management

Surgery
* Adrenalectomy or ovarian cystectomy/oophorectomy.
* Curative in benign lesions.

Adjunctive therapy
* Malignant ovarian and adrenal androgen-secreting tumours are usually resistant to chemotherapy and radiotherapy.

Prognosis

Benign tumours
* Prognosis excellent.
* Hirsutism improves postoperatively, but clitoromegaly, male pattern balding, and deep voice may persist.

Malignant tumours
* *Adrenal tumours* 20% 5 year survival. Most have metastatic disease at the time of surgery.
* *Ovarian tumours* 30% disease-free survival and 40% overall survival at 5 years.

Further reading
Hamilton-Fairley D, Franks S Androgen secreting tumours. In Sheaves R, Jenkins PJ, Wass JAH (ed), *Clinical Endocrine Oncology*. 1997. Oxford: Blackwell Science, pp. 323–329.

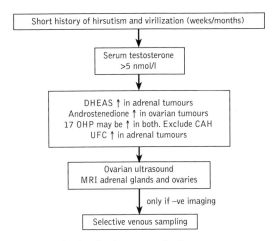

Fig. 56.1 Investigation of androgen-secreting tumours.

Chapter 57
Menstrual disorders – assessment and investigation

Definitions

* *Oligomenorrhoea* is defined as the reduction in the frequency of menses to less than 9 periods a year.
* *Primary amenorrhoea* is the failure of menarche by the age of 16 years.
* *Secondary amenorrhoea* refers to the cessation of menses for >6 months in women who had previously menstruated.

However, the common causes may present with either primary or secondary amenorrhoea.

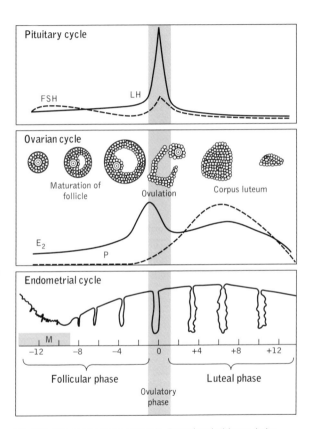

Fig. 57.1 The normal menstrual cycle. Reproduced with permission.

Clinical evaluation

History

- Oestrogen deficiency, e.g. hot flushes, reduced libido and dyspareunia
- Hypothalamic dysregulation, e.g. exercise history, body weight changes, emotional stress or recent physical illness
- Anosmia may indicate Kallman's syndrome
- Hirsutism or acne
- Galactorrhoea
- History suggestive of pituitary, thyroid or adrenal dysfunction
- Drug history – e.g. causes of hyperprolactinaemia.

Physical examination

- Body habitus, e.g. Turner's syndrome, anorexia nervosa
- Breast development and galactorrhoea
- Evidence of hyperandrogenism or hypothyroidism
- Anosmia, visual field defects.

Causes of amenorrhoea

Physiological

- pregnancy and lactation
- postmenopause

Pathological

Primary

- androgen insensitivity syndrome
- congenital absence of uterus
- Turner's syndrome
- Kallman's syndrome

Secondary

- ovarian
  - polycystic ovary syndrome
  - premature ovarian failure
- uterine
  - intrauterine adhesions
- pituitary
  - hyperprolactinaemia
  - hypopituitarism
- hypothalamic
  - weight loss
  - excessive exercise
  - physical or psychological stress
  - craniopharyngioma
  - infiltrative lesions of the hypothalamus.

Investigations

See Fig. 57.2 on facing page.

- Is it primary or secondary ovarian dysfunction?
  - FSH, LH, oestradiol, and prolactin.
- Pelvic ultrasound
  - ovarian and uterine morphology – exclude anatomical abnormalities, polycystic ovary syndrome and Turner's syndrome
  - endometrial thickness – to assess oestrogen status.
- Other tests depending on clinical suspicion
  - serum testosterone in the presence of hyperandrogenism
  - karyotype in primary amenorrhoea or if Turner's syndrome suspected
  - MRI of the pituitary fossa.

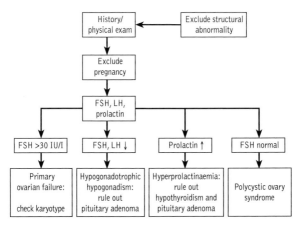

Fig. 57.2 Investigation of amenorrhea.

Management

- Treat underlying disorder, e.g.
  - dopamine agonists for prolactinomas
  - pituitary surgery for pituitary tumours
  - weight gain in anorexia nervosa
- Treat oestrogen deficiency
  - oestrogen/progestogen preparations
- Treat infertility
  - clomiphene in normo-oestrogenic women (e.g. polycystic ovary syndrome)
  - gonadotrophin preparations in oestrogen-deficient women

Further reading

Baird DT Amenorrhoea. *Lancet* 1997; 350: 275–279.

Chapter 58
Premature ovarian failure

Definition

Premature ovarian failure (POF) is a disorder characterized by amenorrhoea, oestrogen deficiency and elevated gonadotropins developing in women <40 years, as a result of loss of ovarian follicular function.

Epidemiology

* Incidence – 0.1% of women <30 years and 1% of those <40 years.
* Accounts for 10% of all cases of secondary amenorrhoea.

Causes of POF
* Chromosomal abnormalities (60%)
  - Turner's syndrome
  - fragile X syndrome
  - other X chromosomal abnormalities
* Gene mutations
  - β subunit of FSH
  - FSH receptor
  - LH receptor
* Autoimmune disease (20%)
* Iatrogenic
  - chemotherapy
  - radiotherapy
* Other
  - galactosaemia
  - enzyme deficiencies, e.g. 17α-hydroxylase deficiency
  - infections, e.g. mumps, HIV, shigella
  - posthysterectomy.

Turner's syndrome (page 631)

* Most common X-chromosome abnormality in females, affecting 1 : 2500 live female births
* Result of complete or partial absence of one X chromosome
* *Clinical features* short stature and gonadal dysgenesis. 90% of affected women have POF.
* *Characteristic phenotype* webbed neck, micrognathia, low-set ears, high arched palate, widely spaced nipples, and cubitus valgus
* *Other associated abnormalities* aortic coarctation and other left sided congenital heart defects, hypothyroidism, osteoporosis, skeletal abnormalities, lymphoedema, congenital renal abnormalities and ENT abnormalities.
* *Diagnosis* lymphocyte karyotype
* *Management in adults:*
  – sex hormone replacement therapy
  – treat complications
* *Follow-up:*
  – baseline renal ultrasound, thyroid autoantibodies
  – annual blood pressure, TFT, lipids, fasting blood glucose
  – 3–5 yearly echocardiogram and bone densitometry.

Pathogenesis

Failure of normal ovarian follicular response to gonadotrophins with consequent failure of ovarian steroidogenesis. POF is the result of either ovarian follicle depletion or failure of the follicles to function (resistant ovary syndrome). May be distinguished by ovarian ultrasound or histologically by ovarian biopsy. Treatment options are the same so invasive techniques looking for the presence of follicles are not indicated.

POF is usually permanent, although women with transient disease have been described. Additionally, <50% of karyotypically normal women with established disease produce oestrogen intermittently and up to a fifth of women may ovulate despite high gonadotrophin levels. Spontaneous pregnancy has been reported in 5%.

Clinical presentation

- *Amenorrhoea*
  - may be primary, particularly in patients with chromosomal abnormalities
- Symptoms of *oestrogen deficiency*
  - not present in those with primary amenorrhoea
  - 75% of women who develop secondary amenorrhoea report hot flushes, night sweats, mood changes, fatigue or dyspareunia; symptoms may precede the onset of menstrual disturbances
- *Autoimmune disease*
  - screen for symptoms and signs of associated autoimmune disorders.
- *Other*
  - past history of radiotherapy, chemotherapy, or pelvic surgery
  - positive family history in a few patients.

Autoimmune diseases and POF

- Responsible for 20% of all cases of POF.
- A second autoimmune disorder is present in 10–40% of women with autoimmune POF:
  - Addison's disease   10%
  - autoimmune thyroid disease   25%
  - type 1 diabetes mellitus   2%
  - myaesthenia gravis   2%
  - SLE also more common.
- POF is present in:
  - 60% of women with autoimmune polyglandular syndrome type 1 (p. 317)
  - 25% of women with autoimmune polyglandular syndrome type 2 (p. 317).
- Steroid cell antibodies are positive in 60–100% of patients with Addison's disease in combination with POF. The presence of positive steroid cell antibodies in women with Addison's disease confers a 40% risk of ultimately developing POF. Other ovarian antibodies have no predictive value.

Investigation

- *Serum gonadotropins*
  - diagnosis is confirmed by serum FSH >40 mIU/L on at least 2 occasions at least 1 month apart
  - disease may have a fluctuating course with high FSH levels returning to normal and later regain of ovulatory function
  - LH also elevated, but FSH usually disproportionately higher than LH.
- *Serum oestradiol* levels are low.
- *Karyotype*
  - all women presenting with primary (hypergonadotropic) amenorrhoea should be karyotyped
  - women with Y chromosomal material should be referred for bilateral gonadectomy to prevent the development of gonadoblastoma. (Testicular feminization, complete androgen resistance.)
- *Pelvic ultrasound* To identify normal ovarian and uterine morphology in women with primary amenorrhoea.
- *Screen for autoimmune disease*
  - thyroid and adrenal cortex autoantibodies; if positive, increases the risk of progression to overt adrenal or thyroid insufficiency
  - ovarian antibodies are of no proven clinical value
  - TSH and fasting blood glucose
  - synacthen test only if adrenal insufficiency is suspected clinically
  - other tests as clinically indicated.
- *Ovarian biopsy* Not indicated.

Annual assessment of women with POF

- Assess adequacy of sex hormone replacement therapy:
  - tolerance and compliance
  - side-effects and complications
  - persistent symptoms of sex hormone deficiency
- Address fertility issues
- Screen for other autoimmune disease (in autoimmune POF):
  - clinical evaluation
  - TSH and fasting blood glucose
  - synacthen test if clinically indicated
- Screen for complications:
  - osteoporosis
  - cardiovascular and cerebrovascular disease.

Management

Sex hormone replacement therapy

• Exogenous oestrogens (HRT) are required to alleviate symptoms and prevent the long-term complications of oestrogen deficiency – osteoporosis and cardiovascular disease. Initial doses depend on the duration of amenorrhoea – if oestrogen deficient for at least 12 months, then start on lowest doses of oestradiol available, to prevent side-effects, but titrate up to full dose within 6 months. If recently amenorrhoeic then full dose may be commenced immediately (see Table 58.1). Doses used in HRT are not contraceptive and do not suppress spontaneous ovarian follicular activity. HRT should be continued at least until the age of 50 years, the mean age of the natural menopause.

• In non-hysterectomized women, a progestagen should be added for 12–14 days a month to prevent endometrial hyperplasia.

• It has been suggested that low-dose androgen replacement therapy may improve persistent fatigue and poor libido despite adequate oestrogen replacement.

Fertility

• A minority of women with POF and a normal karyotype will recover spontaneously. 5% spontaneous fertility rate.

• Oocyte donation and *in vitro* fertilization offer these women their best chance of fertility. Results are promising, with a pregnancy rate of 35% per patient. Results are less good in women with chemotherapy-induced gonadal damage.

• Ovulation induction therapy has been tried but the results have been poor.

• Glucocorticoid therapy has been used in autoimmune POF but efficacy is as yet unknown.

Table 58.1 Hormone replacement therapy in POF

Hormone replacement	Dose
Oestrogen	
Conjugated oestrogen	0.625–1.25 mg daily
Oestradiol valerate	2–4 mg daily
Transdermal oestradiol	100 μg twice a week
Progestagen	12–14 days a month:
Norethisterone	1 mg
Medroxyprogesterone	10 mg
Testosterone	
Intramuscular	50–100 mg every 6–8 months mg/month
Subcutaneous implants	

See section on the menopause (page 405) for full review of hormone replacement therapy.

Prognosis

- Mortality of women with POF is increased twofold.
- Oestrogen deficiency leads to:
  - increased risk of cardiovascular and cerebrovascular disease
  - increased risk of osteoporosis. Up to two-thirds of women with POF and a normal karyotype have reduced BMD, with a z score of −1 or less despite at least intermittent hormone replacement therapy. This may be due to a combination of factors including an initial delay in initiating ERT, poor compliance with ERT and oestrogen 'underdosing'.

Further reading

Barlow DH. Premature ovarian failure. *Baillière's Clinical Obstetrics and Gynaecology* 1996; 10(3): 361–384.

Kalantaridou SN, Davis SR, Nelson LM. Premature ovarian failure. *Endocrinology and Metabolism Clinics of North America* 1998; 27(4): 989–1006.

Chapter 59
Menopause

Definition

• The *menopause* is the permanent cessation of menstruation as a result of ovarian failure and is a retrospective diagnosis made after 12 months of amenorrhoea. The average age of women at the time of the menopause is ~50 years, although smokers reach the menopause ~2 years earlier.

• The *perimenopause* encompasses the menopause transition and the first year following the last menstrual period.

Long-term consequences

• *Osteoporosis* During the perimenopausal period there is an accelerated loss of bone mineral density (BMD), rendering postmenopausal women more susceptible to osteoporotic fractures.

• *Ischaemic heart disease (IHD)* Postmenopausal women are 2–3 times more likely to develop IHD than are premenopausal women, even after age adjustments. The menopause is associated with an increase in risk factors for atherosclerosis, including less favourable lipid profile, decreased insulin sensitivity, and an increased thrombotic tendency.

• *Dementia* Women are 2–3 times more likely to develop Alzheimer's disease than men. It is suggested that oestrogen deficiency may play a role in the development of dementia.

Physiology

The physiology of the menopause remains poorly understood. Ovaries have a finite number of germ cells, with maximal numbers at 20 weeks of intrauterine life. Thereafter, there is a reduction in the number of oocytes until the store is depleted at the time of the menopause. Table 59.1 summarizes hormonal changes during the menopausal transition.

Inhibin B, a peptide produced by the ovarian follicles in response to FSH stimulation, is believed to play a crucial role in the neuroendocrinology of the perimenopause. It is a sensitive indicator of ovarian follicular number and is the earliest marker of ovarian ageing, levels beginning to fall ~12 years before the menopause. Inhibin B acts by suppressing FSH, particularly in the follicular phase of the menstrual cycle. A fall in inhibin B production by failing ovarian follicular cells results in the rise of FSH so characteristic of the menopause. In the early perimenopausal period, FSH levels fluctuate, but the gradual rise in FSH levels maintains oestradiol production by the ovarian follicles. So, contrary to previous belief, average serum oestradiol levels may be high at the onset of the menopause transition, falling only towards the end as the follicles are depleted.

Clinical presentation

There are marked cultural differences in the frequency of symptoms related to the menopause; in particular, vasomotor symptoms and mood disturbances are more commonly reported in western countries.

• *Menstrual disturbances* (90%) Cycles gradually become increasingly anovulatory, and variable in length from about 4 years prior to the menopause. Oligomenorrhoea often precedes permanent amenorrhoea. In 10% of women, menses cease abruptly with no preceding transitional period.

• *Hot flushes* (40%) Often associated with sweats and skin flushing. Highly variable and are thought to be related to fluctuations in oestrogen concentrations. Tend to resolve spontaneously within 5 years of the menopause.

• *Urinary symptoms* (50%) Atrophy of urethral and bladder mucosa after the menopause and decreased sensitivity of a-adrenergic receptors of the bladder neck in the perimenopausal period. This may result in urinary incontinence and an increased risk of urinary tract infections.

• *Sexual dysfunction* (40%) Vaginal atrophy may result in dyspareunia and vaginal dryness. Additionally, falling androgen levels may reduce sexual arousal and libido.

• *Mood changes* (25–50%) Anxiety, forgetfulness, difficulty in concentration and irritability have all been attributed to the menopause. Women with a history of affective disorders are at increased risk of mood disturbances in the perimenopausal period.

Table 59.1 Hormonal changes during the menopausal transition

	Premenopause (from age 36 years)	Early perimenopause	Advanced perimenopause	Menopause
Menstrual cycle	Regular, ovulatory	Irregular, often short cycles, increasingly anovulatory	Oligomenorrhoea	Amenorrhoea
FSH	Rising but within normal range	Intermittently raised, especially in follicular phase	Persistently ↑	↑ ↑
Inhibin B	Declining	Low	Low	Very low
E₂	Normal	Normal	Normal/low	Low

Evaluation (e.g. if HRT is being considered)

- *History:*
  - perimenopausal symptoms and their severity
  - assess risk factors for cardiovascular disease and osteoporosis
  - assess risk factors for breast cancer and thromboembolic disease
  - history of active liver disease
- *Examination:*
  - blood pressure
  - breasts
  - pelvic examination, including cervical smear
- *Investigations:*
  - *FSH* levels fluctuate markedly in perimenopausal period and correlate poorly with symptoms. Remember, a raised FSH in the perimenopausal period may not necessarily indicate infertility, so contraception, if desired, should continue until the menopause
  - *mammography* indicated prior to starting oestrogen replacement therapy only in high risk women; otherwise, mammography should be offered as per national screening programme
  - *endometrial biopsy* does not need to be performed routinely, but is essential in women with abnormal uterine bleeding.

Hormone replacement therapy

The aims of treatment of perimenopausal women are twofold:

- alleviation of menopausal symptoms
- preventing the long-term consequences of oestrogen deficiency.

Alleviation of symptoms

- *Hot flushes* Respond very well to oestrogen therapy in a dose-dependent manner. High doses may be required initially (up to the equivalent of 2.5 mg conjugated oestrogens), particularly in younger women or in those whose symptoms develop abruptly. Reduce dose gradually.

Alternative treatment (e.g. in those with a contraindication to HRT, or intolerant of it): megestrol acetate in a dose of 20 mg 2× daily reduces hot flushes by up to 70%. Main side-effect is weight gain. Clonidine is less effective, reducing the occurrence of flushes by 20%, and its use is limited by side-effects. Venlataxine may be useful.

- *Urinary symptoms* A trial of HRT, local or systemic, may improve stress and urge incontinence as well as the frequency of cystitis.
- *Vaginal atrophy* Systemic or local oestrogen therapy improves vaginal dryness and dyspareunia. A maximum of 6 months' use is recommended unless combined with a progestagen as systemic absorption may increase the risk of endometrial hyperplasia. If oestrogens are contraindicated, then vaginal moisturizers, e.g. Replens, may help.
- *Mood disturbances* HRT may improve psychological well-being and mood.

Prevention of long-term consequences of oestrogen deficiency

Cardiovascular disease

HRT users have a lower age-adjusted all-cause mortality compared with non-users, primarily as a result of the reduction in IHD risk. Studies have shown that the risk of IHD is reduced by up to 50% in women receiving HRT.

HRT reduces risk factors for IHD (see Table 59.2). However, recent evidence suggests that HRT may not be beneficial for secondary prevention of IHD and may actually increase morbidity in the year following a myocardial infarction.

Osteoporosis

HRT has been shown to increase bone mineral density in the lumbar spine by 3–5% and at the femoral neck by about 2%, by inhibiting bone resorption. There is an associated 50% reduction in fracture risk, protection being highest in women on HRT for at least 10 years. Timing of initiation of treatment in order to achieve maximal bone protection remains controversial. Evidence suggests that initiation of HRT soon after the menopause is associated with the lowest hip fracture risk, but discontinuation of HRT results in bone loss to pretreatment levels.

Women at increased risk of osteoporosis may therefore be offered HRT to prevent bone loss and osteoporotic fractures. This may be initiated at the time of the menopause or alternatively deferred until the time when fracture risk is greatest, i.e. age 65 years and over.

Alzheimer's disease

Recent evidence suggests that the risk of developing Alzheimer's disease is reduced by up to 50% in women receiving HRT. In women with established Alzheimer's disease, cognitive function may improve if HRT is started and disease progression is delayed by up to 2 years. Protection is maximal with higher doses of oestrogen and longer durations of treatment. In postmenopausal women without dementia, HRT may also improve cognitive function. Mechanisms are unknown but it is thought that oestrogens may improve cerebral perfusion and afford neuronal protection.

Further research is required but it may be prudent to recommend HRT in women at risk of dementia, e.g. family history of Alzheimer's disease. Additionally, a trial of HRT may help women with established disease.

Colorectal cancer

Preliminary research suggests that the rates of colorectal cancer are 50% lower in current users of HRT. However, more research is required before recommending HRT to prevent this disease.

Risks of HRT

Table 59.3 summarizes contraindications to HRT.

Breast cancer

- *No personal or family history of breast cancer* 30% increased risk of breast cancer after 10 years of HRT. Risk is not related to HRT type, only to duration of use. The risk is increased by 2.3% per year of use. Risk is reduced to that of general population 5 years after discontinuing HRT. Mortality is not increased in breast cancer developing in women on HRT.

Side-effects commonly associated with HRT

- *Breast tenderness* usually subsides within 4–6 months of use. If troublesome, use lower oestrogen dose and increase gradually.
- *Mood changes* commonly associated with progestin therapy; manage by changing dose or preparation of progestin.
- *Irregular vaginal bleeding* may be a problem in women on a continuous combined preparation; usually subsides after 6–12 months of treatment. Spotting persists in 10% – may change to a cyclic preparation.

Table 59.2 Effects of HRT on IHD risk factors

Risk factor	Effect of HRT
Lipids	
HDL	↑
LDL	↓
Triglycerides	↑ (transdermal oestrogens have no effect on triglycerides)
Fasting glucose and insulin	↓ (postprandial levels are unchanged)
Fibrinogen	↓
Arterial blood pressure	Unchanged
Obesity	HRT does not cause weight gain
Endothelial function	Endothelial-dependent vasodilatation is enhanced, possibly by increasing nitric oxide production

Current recommendations for the institution of HRT in women for IHD prevention

- *women at high risk of IHD but no clinical disease*
  HRT recommended
- *women with a history of a coronary event*
  initiation of HRT probably not recommended, but may be continued in women already receiving it.

Table 59.3 Contraindications to HRT

Absolute	Relative – seek advice
Undiagnosed vaginal bleeding	Past history of endometrial cancer
Pregnancy	Family or past history of thromboembolism
Active DVT	Active liver disease
Active endometrial cancer	Hypertriglyceridaemia
Breast cancer	

- *Family history of breast cancer* Risk of breast cancer may be increased fourfold as a result of the family history, but there is little evidence that the risk is increased further by the use of HRT. May use HRT in these women if strong indications exist after explaining above risks.

- *Past history of breast cancer* Avoid HRT. If patient is very troubled with vasomotor symptoms and the breast cancer is cured with good prognostic factors, then short-term HRT may be considered as long as patient understands risks. Studies are underway looking at the use of HRT in women with history of breast cancer.

- *Benign breast disease* HRT does not increase the risk of breast cancer.

Venous thromboembolism

- *Low-risk women* Up to fourfold increased risk of deep vein thrombosis (DVT) in HRT users. Absolute risk remains small – 30/100 000 women.

- *Family history of DVT* Do thrombophilia screen. If positive, then avoid HRT. Women with a positive family history of thromboembolism are still at a slightly increased risk themselves even if the results of the thrombophilia screen are negative.

- *Past history of DVT/PE* Risk of recurrence is 5% per year so avoid HRT unless on long-term warfarin therapy.

Endometrial cancer

No increased risk in women taking combined oestrogen/progestin preparations. Women with cured stage I tumours may safely take HRT.

Gallstones

Risk of gallstones is increased twofold in HRT users.

Migraine

Migraines may increase in severity and frequency in HRT users. A trial of HRT is still worthwhile if indications are present. Modification in the dose of oestrogen or its preparation may improve symptoms. Avoid conjugated oestrogens as these are most commonly associated with an increase in the frequency of migraines.

Endometriosis and uterine fibroids

The risk of recurrence of endometriosis or of growth of uterine fibroids is low on HRT.

Liver disease

Use parenteral oestrogens to avoid hepatic metabolism and monitor liver function

Phytoestrogens

Phytoestrogens have not been shown to improve menopausal symptoms. Some data suggest a cardioprotective effect and protection against bone loss, although further work is required. The effect on breast cancer is unclear.

HRT regimens

Oestrogen preparations

In younger, symptomatic, often perimenopausal women, higher doses of oestrogen are often required initially, which can be reduced gradually to the recommended bone-conserving doses shown in Table 59.4.

Older women who have been amenorrhoeic for over a year often do not tolerate the introduction of the recommended dose of oestrogen. The lowest possible dose of oestrogen should therefore be used initially and the dose gradually built up over 6 months.

Route of administration

* *Oral route* is the most popular. Disadvantages:
  - first pass hepatic metabolism means that plasma oestrogen levels are variable, so symptoms do not always respond
  - may be associated with nausea and may exacerbate liver disease
  - must be taken daily so there is no breakthrough of symptoms
* *Transdermal patches* avoid first pass effect and are thus ideal in women with liver disease or hypertriglyceridaemia. Additionally, patches provide constant systemic hormone levels. However, 10% of women develop skin reactions. Try to avoid moisture and to rotate patch sites to prevent this.
* *Gels* have the advantages of patches but skin irritation is less common.
* *Subcutaneous implants* have the advantage of good compliance. However, if side-effects develop, implants are difficult to remove. Additionally, may release oestradiol for up to 3 years after insertion and cyclical progestagens must be given until oestrogen levels are not detectable.

Progestagen preparations

See Table 59.5 Must be added in non-hysterectomized women to avoid endometrial hyperplasia and subsequent carcinoma.

Sequential cyclical regimen

Give progestagen for a minimum of 10 days a month. Usually given for the first 12 days of each calendar month. Quarterly regimen available – progestagen given for 14 days four times a year. However, the risk of endometrial hyperplasia on such a regimen is unknown.

90% of women have a monthly withdrawal bleed. 10% may be amenorrhoeic with no harmful consequences. Bleeding should start after the 9th day of progestagen therapy.

Continuous combined regimen

Lower doses of progestagen are given on a daily basis. Uterine bleeding is usually light in amount but timing is unpredictable. Bleeding

Table 59.4 Oestrogen presparations

Preparation	Dose
Conjugated oestrogens (PO)	0.625–1.25 mg daily
Oestradiol valerate (PO)	2 mg daily
Oestradiol transdermal patch	100 µg twice a week. New patch twice a week
Oestradiol gel	1–1.5 mg daily
Oestradiol subcutaneous implant	25–100 mg every 4–8 months. Check serum E_2 prior to implant

Table 59.5 Dosage of progestagen presparations

Progestin	Cyclical dose (d1–12)	Continuous daily dose
Medroxyprogesterone acetate (least androgenic)	10 mg	2.5–5 mg (higher dose reduces bleeding)
Dydrogesterone	10 mg	Unknown
Norgestrel	150 µg	Unknown
Norethisterone (most androgenic)	0.7–1 mg	0.35–1 mg

Who and how to investigate for irregular uterine bleeding

- *Sequential cyclical HRT* 3 or more cycles of: bleeding before the 9th day of progestagen therapy or change in the duration or intensity of uterine bleeding.
- *Continuous combined HRT* In first 12 months if bleeding is heavy or extended, if it continues after 12 months of use, or if it starts after a period of amenorrhoea.
- *Endometrial assessment* Essential in women with irregular uterine bleeding. Vaginal ultrasound, looking at endometrial thickness, is a sensitive method of detecting endometrial disease. Endometrial thickness of <5 mm excludes disease in 96–99% of cases, a sensitivity similar to that of endometrial biopsy. However, specificity is poor so if the endometrium is >5 mm (as it will be in 50% of postmenopausal women on HRT) endometrial biopsy will be required to rule out carcinoma.

should stop in 90% of women within 12 months, the majority in 6 months.

Ideal for older women who do not want monthly withdrawal bleeds. Contraindicated in perimenopausal women, as irregular uterine bleeding is more likely and difficult to assess.

Tibolone (2.5 mg a day)

A synthetic steroid with mixed oestrogenic, progestogenic and weak androgenic activities. An alternative form of HRT which does not induce uterine bleeding. It is protective against osteoporosis but its effects on the cardiovascular system are unknown.

Androgen replacement therapy

- *Indications* Poor well-being and libido despite HRT. Studies suggest that low dose testosterone replacement therapy may enhance libido in addition to improving mood.

- *Mode of administration* Subcutaneous testosterone implants 50–100 mg every 6–8 months. No other androgen preparation currently available in the UK in doses suitable for women.

- *Side-effects and possible complications* Virilization has been reported in over a third of women. Adverse changes to lipid profile commonly occur.

Further reading

Greendale GA, Lee NP, Arriola ER. The menopause. *Lancet* 1999; 353: 571–580.

Johnson SR. The clinical decision regarding hormone replacement therapy. *Endocrinology and Metabolism Clinics of North America* 1997; 26(2): 413–434.

Prior JC. Perimenopause: the complex endocrinology of the menopausal transition. *Endocrine Reviews* 1998; 19(4): 397–428.

Chapter 60
Combined oral contraceptive pill

- *Ethinyl oestradiol (EE2)*
  - standard dose is 30 μg, but in older women or those with possible cardiovascular risk factors, 20 μg EE2 may be appropriate
  - 50 μg of EE2 may be indicated in patients on antiepileptic medication.
- *Progestagen* Commonly used oral contraceptive pills (OCPs) contain second-generation progestagens such as *levonorgestrel* (0.15–0.25 mg) and *norethisterone* (1 mg). OCPs containing third-generation progestagens (e.g. *gestodene* and *desogestrel*) are now less commonly used because of the increased risk of thromboembolism.

OCP side-effects

* low mood
* nausea
* fluid retention and weight gain
* breast tenderness and enlargement
* headache
* reduced libido
* chloasma

OCP preparation

* *1st generation*
  - Norynyl-1
  - Ovran
* *2nd generation*
  - Bi Novum
  - Brevinor
  - Cilest
  - Eugynon 30
  - Loestrin 20/30
  - Logynon
  - Microgynon 30/30 ED
  - Norimin
  - Ovran 30
  - Ovranette
  - Ovysmen
  - Synphase
  - Trinordiol
  - Tri Novum
* *3rd generation*
  - Femodene/ED
  - Femodette
  - Marvelon
  - Marvelon
  - Mercilon
  - Triadene
  - Tri Minulet

Risks

Venous thromboembolism

- The risk of venous thromboembolism in non-pregnant women (5 per 100 000 women/year) is increased threefold in women on the OCP, particularly in obese women.
- Women with a family history of thromboembolism should undergo a thrombophilia screen before starting the OCP.

Arterial thrombosis

- There is an increased risk of developing IHD in women over the age of 35 years who are on the OCP. The risk is further increased tenfold in smokers.
- The relative risk of ischaemic or haemorrhagic stroke is only slightly increased in women over the age of 35 years, but not in younger women.
- Risk of either arterial or venous thrombosis returns to normal within 3 months of discontinuing the OCP.

Hypertension

May be caused by the OCP, and if already present, may be more resistant to treatment.

Hepatic disease

Raised hepatic enzymes may be seen in women on the OCP.
The incidence of benign hepatic tumours is also increased.

Gallstones

The risk of developing gallstones is slightly increased by taking the OCP (RR = 1.2).

Breast cancer

- There is a slightly increased risk of breast cancer developing before the age of 36 years in women using the OCP (RR = 1.3), particularly in those who began taking the OCP in their teens.
- The risk does not seem to be related to the duration of exposure to the OCP nor to the EE2 dose.
- The relative risk of developing breast cancer returns to normal 10 years after discontinuing the OCP.

Thrombophilia screen

antithrombin III
protein C
protein S
factor V Leiden

Table 60.1 OCP contraindications

Absolute	Relative
History of heart disease – ischaemic or valvular	Migraine
Pulmonary hypertension	Sickle-cell disease
History of arterial or venous thrombosis	Gallstones
History of cerebrovascular disease	Inflammatory bowel disease
High risk of thrombosis, e.g. factor V Leiden, antiphospholipid antibodies	Hypertension
Liver disease	Hyperlipidaemia
Migraine if severe or associated with focal aura	Diabetes mellitus
Breast or genital tract cancer	Obesity
Pregnancy	Smokers
Presence of two or more relative contraindications	
Age over 35 years	Otosclerosis
	Family history of thrombosis
	Family history of breast cancer

Consider using a progesterone-only pill in women with contraindications to the combined OCP.

Practical issues

Age and the OCP

- Women with no risk factors for arterial or venous thrombosis may continue to use the combined OCP until the age of 50 years.
- Those with risk factors for thromboembolism and IHD should avoid the OCP after the age of 35 years.
- All women on the OCP after the age of 35 years should be on the lowest effective oestrogen dose (e.g. 20 μg EE2).
- Contraception after the menopause: assume fertile for the first year after last menstrual period if >50 years.

Breakthrough bleeding

Causes include:

- genital tract disease
- insufficient oestrogen dose
- inappropriate progestagen
- missed pill
- taking two packets continuously
- gastroenteritis
- drug interactions, e.g. antibiotics, hepatic enzyme inducers

Antibiotics and the OCP

Broad-spectrum antibiotics interfere with intestinal flora, thereby reducing bioavailability of the OCP. Additional methods of contraception should be used.

OCP and surgery

- Stop OCP at least 4 weeks before major surgery and any surgery to the legs. Do not restart until fully mobile for at least 2 weeks.
- If emergency surgery, then stop OCP and start antithrombotic prophylaxis.

Chapter 61
Testicular physiology

Anatomy

- Normal adult male testicular volume 15–30 ml.
- Testicular temperature 2°C lower than rest of body because of scrotal location. This is necessary for normal spermatogenesis.
- Two main units with differing functions:
  - *Interstitial cells* Comprised of Leydig cells which are found in between the seminiferous tubules and close to the blood vessels. Produce testosterone.
  - *Seminiferous tubules* Make up 90% of testicular volume. Spermatogenesis occurs here, in the presence of high intratesticular concentrations of testosterone. Made up of *germ cells* and *Sertoli cells*. Sertoli cells support spermatogenesis and secrete various hormones, including inhibin and in the embryo, Mullerian inhibitory factor. The former inhibits FSH secretion from the pituitary gland and the latter is responsible for suppressing female sex organ development during sexual differentiation *in utero*.

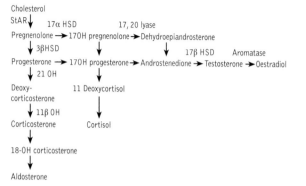

Fig. 61.1 Testosterone biosynthesis pathway. StAR, steroidogenic autoregulatory protein; 3βHSD, 3β-hydroxydehydrogenase; 21 OH, 21-hydroxylase; 17α OH, 17α-hydroxylase; 11β OH, 11β-hydroxylase.

Regulation of testicular function

Regulation of androgen production

Hypothalamic hormones

- *Gonadotropin releasing hormone (GnRH)* is secreted by the hypothalamus in a pulsatile manner in response to stimuli from the cerebral cortex and limbic system via various neurotransmitters, e.g. endorphins, catecholamines and dopamine and testicular feedback systems.
- GnRH release initially occurs during sleep in early puberty and then throughout the day in adulthood. It stimulates the secretion of *luteinizing hormone* (LH) and *follicle stimulating hormone* (FSH) by the pituitary gland. The pattern of GnRH secretion is crucial for normal gonadotrophin secretion. Faster pulse frequencies are essential for LH secretion whereas slower frequences favour FSH secretion. Continuous administration of GnRH abolishes both LH and FSH secretion.

Pituitary hormones

- LH binds to Leydig cell receptors and stimulates the synthesis and secretion of testosterone.
- FSH binds to Sertoli cell receptors and stimulates the production of seminiferous tubule fluid as well as a number of substances thought to be important for spermatogenesis.
- Their secretion is regulated by GnRH pulses and through negative feedback from testicular hormones and peptides.

Testis

- Testosterone is the main androgen produced by the Leydig cells of the testis. Small amounts of androstenedione, dehydroepiandrostenedione (DHEA), and dihydrotestosterone (DHT) are also produced. Testosterone has a circadian rhythm with maximum secretion at around 8 a.m. and minimum around 9 p.m.
- Small amounts of oestradiol are also produced in the testis, by the conversion from testosterone. However, most of the circulating oestradiol in males occurs as a result of aromatization of androgens in adipose tissue.
- FSH, in the presence of adequate testosterone levels, stimulates the secretion of inhibin by Sertoli cells. This in turn acts as a potent inhibitor of FSH secretion.

- The secretion of pituitary gonadotrophins is tightly regulated by testicular function. LH secretion is inhibited by testosterone and its metabolites whereas FSH secretion is controlled by both inhibin and testosterone. High concentrations of testosterone or of inhibin results in a negative feedback inhibition of FSH secretion (see Fig. 61.2).

- Testicular function is also under paracrine control. Inhibin and insulin-like growth factor-1 (IGF-1) act with LH to enhance testosterone production, whereas cytokines inhibit Leydig cell function.

Regulation of spermatogenesis

See Fig. 61.2.

- Both FSH and LH are required for the initiation of spermatogenesis at puberty. LH, by stimulating Leydig cell activity, plays an important part in the early phases of sperm production, when high intratesticular concentrations of testosterone are essential. FSH through its action on the Sertoli cells, is vital for sperm maturation.

- The whole process of spermatogenesis takes approximately 74 days, followed by another 12–21 days for sperm transport through the epididymis. This means that events which may affect spermatogenesis may not be apparent for up to 3 months.

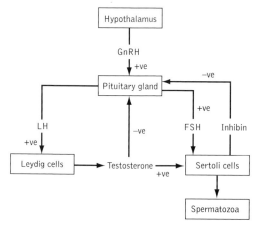

Fig. 61.2 Regulation of spematogenesis.

Physiology

Testosterone transport

+ 2–4% of circulating testosterone is free and therefore biologically active. The rest is bound to proteins, particularly albumin and sex hormone binding globulin (SHBG).

Testosterone metabolism

+ Testosterone is converted in target tissues to the more potent androgen DHT in the presence of the enzyme 5α reductase. There are multiple 5α-reductase isoenzymes; type 2 is the isoenzyme responsible for DHT synthesis in the genitalia, genital skin and hair follicles. It is therefore essential for normal male virilization and sexual development.

+ Both testosterone and DHT exert their activity by binding to androgen receptors, the latter more avidly than testosterone. The androgen receptor is encoded by a gene found on the long arm of the X chromosome (Xq).

+ Testosterone may alternatively be converted into oestradiol through the action of the aromatase enzyme, found in greatest quantities in adipose tissue.

+ Testosterone and its metabolites are inactivated in the liver and excreted in the urine.

Androgen action

+ male sexual differentiation during embryogenesis
+ development and maintenance of male secondary sex characteristics after puberty
+ normal male sexual function and behaviour
+ spermatogenesis
+ regulation of gonadotropin secretion.

Chapter 62
Male hypogonadism

Definition

Failure of testes to produce adequate amounts of testosterone, spermatozoa, or both.

Epidemiology

- Klinefelter's syndrome is the most common congenital cause and is thought to occur with an incidence of 1 : 500 live births.
- Acquired hypogonadism is even more common, affecting up to 20% of males.

Evaluation of male hypogonadism
Presentation
* failure to progress through puberty
* erectile dysfunction
* infertility.

The clinical presentation depends on:
* the age of onset (congenital vs acquired)
* the severity (complete vs partial)
* the duration (functional vs permanent).

Secondary hypogonadism

Definition

Hypogonadism as a result of hypothalamic or pituitary dysfunction.

Diagnosis

- low 9 a.m. serum testosterone
- normal/low LH and FSH.

Causes

Kallmann's syndrome

A genetic disorder characterized by failure of episodic GnRH secretion ± anosmia. Results from disordered migration of GnRH-producing neurons into the hypothalamus.

Epidemiology

- incidence of 1 in 10 000 males
- male : female ratio = 4 :1.

Diagnosis

- anosmia in 75%
- increased risk of cleft lip and palate, sensorineural deafness, cerebellar ataxia, and renal agenesis.
- low testosterone, LH, and FSH levels
- normal rest of pituitary function
- normal MRI pituitary gland and hypothalamus; absent olfactory bulbs may be seen on MRI
- normalization of pituitary and gonadal function in response to physiological GnRH replacement.

Genetics

- most commonly a result of an isolated gene mutation
- may be inherited in an X-linked, autosomal dominant, or recessive trait
- *KAL* gene defect responsible for some cases of Kallmann's syndrome is located on Xp22.3
- 12–15% incidence of delayed puberty in families of subjects with Kallmann's syndrome compared with 1% general population.

Causes of secondary hypogonadism

- Idiopathic
  - Kallmann's
  - idiopathic hypogonadotrophic hypogonadism (IHH)
  - fertile eunuch syndrome
  - congenital adrenal hypoplasia
- Functional
  - exercise
  - weight changes
  - anabolic steroids
  - stress – physical/psychological
  - systemic illness
  - medication and recreational drugs
  - infiltrative disorders, e.g. sarcoidosis, haemochromatosis
  - head trauma
  - radiotherapy
  - surgery to the pituitary gland or hypothalamus
- Miscellaneous
  - haemochromatosis
  - Prader–Willi syndrome (p. 431)
  - Laurence–Moon–Biedl syndrome (p. 431)

Management

* androgen replacement therapy.
* when fertility is desired, testosterone is stopped and exogenous gonadotropins are administered (see p. 477).

Idiopathic hypogonadotrophic hypogonadism (IHH)

* Congenital form is indistinguishable from Kallmann's syndrome apart from the absence of anosmia. Over 90% of patients are male.
* GnRH receptor gene mutation is an uncommon cause of IHH.
* Men with acquired IHH may go through normal puberty and have normal testicular size, but present with infertility or poor libido and potency. May be temporary, with normalization of gonadal function after stopping GnRH or testosterone therapy.

Fertile eunuch syndrome

* Incomplete GnRH deficiency. Enough to maintain normal spermatogenesis and testicular growth but insufficient for adequate virilization.
* May require testosterone/hCG for fertility.

Congenital adrenal hypoplasia

* Rare X-linked or autosomal recessive disease caused by a mutation of the *DAX* gene, which is located on the X chromosome.
* Presents with primary adrenal failure in infancy.
* Hypothalamic hypogonadism is also present.

Structural

* Usually associated with other pituitary hormonal deficiencies.
* In children, craniopharyngiomas are the most common cause. Cranial irradiation for leukaemia or brain tumours may also result in secondary hypogonadism.
* The commonest lesions in adulthood are prolactinomas.

Systemic illness

* Severe illness of any kind may cause hypogonadotropic hypogonadism (see table).

Drugs

* Anabolic steroids, cocaine and narcotic drugs may all result in secondary hypogonadism
* All drugs causing hyperprolactinaemia (see p. 137) will also cause hypogonadism.

Systemic illness resulting in hypogonadism

* Secondary hypogonadism
  – any acute illness (e.g. myocardial infarction, sepsis, head injury)
  – severe stress
  – haemochromatosis
  – endocrine disease (Cushing's syndrome, hyperprolactinaemia)
* Primary hypogonadism
  – liver cirrhosis
  – chronic renal failure
  – chronic anaemia (thalassaemia major, sickle cell disease)
  – gastrointestinal disease (coeliac disease, Crohn's disease)
  – AIDS
  – rheumatological disease (rheumatoid arthritis)
  – respiratory disease (e.g. chronic obstructive airways disease, cystic fibrosis)
  – cardiac disease (e.g. congestive cardiac failure)

Prader–Willi syndrome

* A congenital syndrome caused by deletion of part of paternally derived chromosome 15q which is characterized by severe obesity, mental retardation, and hypogonadotropic hypogonadism.

Laurence–Moon–Biedl syndrome

* Congenital syndrome characterized by severe obesity, gonadotropin deficiency, retinitis pigmentosa, polydactyly, and mental retardation.

Primary hypogonadism

Due to testicular failure

Diagnosis

* low 9 a.m. serum testosterone
* elevated LH and FSH.

Causes

Genetic

Klinefelter's syndrome

The most common congenital form of primary hypogonadism, affecting approximately 1 : 500 men.

* Clinical manifestations
  - reduced testicular volume
  - gynaecomastia
  - eunuchoidism
  - intellectual dysfunction in 40%
  - NB 20 times increased risk of breast carcinoma.
* Diagnosis
  - karyotyping – 47,XXY or 46,XY/47,XXY mosaicism
  - low testosterone, elevated LH and FSH
  - elevated SHBG and oestradiol
  - azoospermia.
* Management
  - androgen replacement
  - NB Unlikely to normalize gonadotrophins.

Other chromosomal disorders

XX males

  - Due to an X to Y translocation with only a part of the Y present in one of the X chromosomes.
  - Incidence 1 : 10 000 births.
  - Similar clinical and biochemical features to Klinefelter's syndrome. In addition, short stature and hypospadias may be present.

XX/X0 (mixed gonadal dysgenesis)

– Occasionally phenotypically male with hypospadias and intra-abdominal dysgenetic gonads.

– Bilateral gonadectomy is essential because of the risk of neoplasia, followed by androgen replacement therapy.

XYY syndrome

– Taller than average, but often have primary gonadal failure with impaired spermatogenesis.

Y chromosome deletions

– Causes oligo/azoospermia. Testosterone levels are not usually affected.

Noonan's syndrome

– 46,XY karyotype and male external genitalia. However, several stigmata of Turner's syndrome (short stature, webbed neck, ptosis, low set ears, lymphoedema) and increased risk of right-sided cardiac anomalies. Most have cryptorchidism and primary testicular failure.

Cryptorchidism

♦ 10% of male neonates have undescended testes, but most of these will descend into the scrotum eventually, so that the incidence of postpubertal cryptorchidism is less than 0.5%.

♦ 15% of cases have bilateral cryptorchidism.

Consequences

♦ 75% of males with bilateral cryptorchidism are infertile.

♦ 10% risk of testicular malignancy, highest risk in those with intra-abdominal testes.

♦ Low testosterone and raised gonadotropins in bilateral cryptorchidism.

Treatment

♦ *Orchidopexy* Best performed before 18 months, certainly before age 5 years.

♦ *Gonadectomy* In patients with intra-abdominal testes, followed by androgen replacement.

Orchitis

♦ 25% of males who develop mumps after puberty have associated orchitis and 25–50% of these will develop primary testicular failure.

♦ HIV infection may also be associated with orchitis.

♦ Primary testicular failure may occur as part of an autoimmune disease.

Chemotherapy and radiotherapy

• Cytotoxic drugs, particularly alkylating agents, are gonadotoxic. Infertility occurs in 50% of patients following chemotherapy for most malignancies, and a significant number of men require androgen replacement therapy because of low testosterone levels.

• The testes are radiosensitive so hypogonadism can occur as a result of scattered radiation during the treatment of Hodgkin's dosease, for example.

• If fertility is desired, sperm should be cryopreserved prior to cancer therapy.

Other drugs

• Sulfasalazine, colchicine and statins may all affect testicular function.

• Alcohol excess will also cause primary testicular failure.

Chronic illness

• Any chronic illness may affect testicular function, in particular chronic renal failure, liver cirrhosis, and haemochromatosis.

Varicocoele

• A debatable cause of primary hypogonadism.

Testicular trauma

• Testicular torsion is another common cause of loss of a testis, and it may also affect the function of the remaining testis.

Testicular dysfunction: clinical characteristics of male hypogonadism

Testicular failure occurring before onset of puberty

- testicular volume <5 ml
- penis <5 cm long
- lack of scrotal pigmentation and rugae
- gynaecomastia
- high-pitched voice
- central fat distribution
- eunuchoidism:
  - arm span 1 cm greater than height
  - lower segment > upper segment
- delayed bone age
- no male escutcheon
- decreased body and facial hair.

Testicular failure occurring after puberty

- testes soft, volume <15 ml
- normal penile length
- normal skeletal proportions
- gynaecomastia
- normal male hair distribution but reduced amount
- osteoporosis.

Clinical assessment

History

- *Developmental history* congenital urinary tract abnormalities, e.g. hypospadias, late testicular descent or cryptorchidism
- *Delayed or incomplete puberty*
- *Infections* e.g. mumps, orchitis
- *Abdominal/genital trauma*
- *Testicular torsion*
- *Anosmia*
- *Drug history* e.g. sulfasalazine, antihypertensives, chemotherapy, cimetidine, radiotherapy; alcohol and recreational drugs also important.
- *General medical history* Chronic illness, particularly respiratory, neurological and cardiac.
- *Gynaecomastia* Common (see p. 446) during adolescence. Recent onset gynaecomastia in adulthood – must rule out oestrogen-producing tumour.
- *Family history* Young's syndrome (p. 472), cystic fibrosis, Kallman's syndrome.
- *Sexual history* Erectile function, frequency of intercourse, sexual techniques. Absence of morning erections suggests an organic cause of erectile dysfunction.

Physical examination

- body hair distribution
- muscle mass and fat distribution
- eunuchoidism
- gynaecomastia
- genital examination:
  - *pubic hair* normal male escutcheon
  - *phallus* normal >5 cm length and >3 cm width
  - *testes* size and consistency (normal >15 ml and firm)
    - look for nodules or areas of tenderness
- general examination
  - look for evidence of systemic disease
  - assess sense of smell and visual fields.

Hormonal evaluation of testicular function

Serum testosterone

Diurnal variation in circulating testosterone, peak levels occurring in the early morning. 30% variation between highest and lowest testosterone levels, so 9 a.m. plasma testosterone essential. If level is low, this should be repeated.

Sex hormone binding globulin (SHBG)

* Only 2–4% of circulating testosterone is unbound. 50% is bound to SHBG and the rest to albumin.
* Concentrations of SHBG should be taken into account when interpreting a serum testosterone result. SHBG levels may be affected by a variety of conditions (see table 62.1).

Gonadotrophins

Raised FSH and LH in primary testicular failure and inappropriately low in pituitary or hypothalamic hypogonadism. Should always exclude hyperprolactinaemia in secondary hypogonadism.

Oestradiol

Results from the conversion of testosterone and androstenedione by aromatase. See table 62.2 for causes of an elevated oestradiol. Request serum oestradiol level if gynaecomastia is present or a testicular tumour is suspected.

hCG stimulation test

* Diagnostic test for examining Leydig cell function.
* hCG 2000 iu i/m given on days 0 and 2; testosterone measured on days 0,2, and 4.
* In prepubertal boys with absent scrotal testes, a response to hCG indicates intra-abdominal testes. Failure of testosterone to rise after hCG suggests absence of functioning testicular tissue. An exaggerated response to hCG is seen in secondary hypogonadism.

Clomiphene stimulation test

* Used to assess the integrity of the hypothalamo–pituitary testicular axis.
* A normal response to 3 mg/kg (max 200 mg) clomiphene daily for 7 days is a twofold increase in LH and FSH measured on days 0,4,7, and 10.
* Subnormal response indicates hypothalamic or pituitary hypogonadism but does not differentiate between the two.

Table 62.1 Factors affecting SHBG concentrations

Raised SHBG	Low SHBG
Androgen deficiency	Hyperinsulinaemia
GH deficiency	Obesity
Ageing	Acromegaly
Thyrotoxicosis	Androgen treatment
Oestrogens	Hypothyroidism
Liver cirrhosis	Cushing's syndrome/glucocorticoid therapy
	Nephrotic syndrome

Table 62.2 Causes of raised oestogens in men

Neoplasia
testicular
adrenal
hepatoma
Primary testicular failure
Liver disease
Thyrotoxicosis
Obesity
Androgen resistance syndromes
Antiandrogen therapy.

Chapter 63
Androgen replacement therapy

Treatment aims

- *Improve libido and sexual function* Testosterone replacement therapy will induce virilization in the hypogonadal male and restores libido and erectile function.
- *Improve mood and well-being* Most studies show an improvement in mood and well-being following testosterone replacement therapy.
- *Improve muscle mass and strength* Testosterone has direct anabolic effects on skeletal muscle and has been shown to increase muscle mass and strength when given to hypogonadal men. Lean body mass is also increased with a reduction in fat mass.
- *Prevent osteoporosis* Hypogonadism is a risk factor for osteoporosis. Testosterone inhibits bone resorption, thereby reducing bone turnover. Its administration to hypogonadal men has been shown to improve bone mineral density and reduce the risk of developing osteoporosis.
- NB *Fertility* is not restored by androgen replacement therapy. Men with secondary hypogonadism who desire fertility may be treated with gonadotropins to initiate and maintain spermatogenesis (see p. 477). Prior testosterone therapy will not affect fertility prospects but should be stopped before initiating gonadotropin treatment. Men with primary hypogonadism will not respond to gonadotropin or GnRH therapy.

Indications for treatment

Male hypogonadism of any cause

Table 63.1 Contraindications to androgen replacement therapy

Absolute	Relative
Prostate cancer	Benign prostate hyperplasia
Breast cancer	Polycythaemia
	Sleep apnoea

Pretreatment evaluation

Clinical evaluation

History or symptoms of:
- prostatic hypertrophy
- breast or prostate cancer
- cardiovascular disease
- sleep apnoea.

Examination
- rectal examination of prostate
- breasts

Laboratory evaluation
- prostatic specific antigen (PSA) (NB PSA is often low in hypogonadal men, rising to normal age-matched levels with androgen replacement.)
- haemoglobin and haematocrit
- serum lipids

Monitoring of therapy

3 months after initiating therapy and then 6–12 monthly:
- clinical evaluation
- serum testosterone
- rectal examination of the prostate
- PSA (if>45 years)
- haemoglobin and haematocrit
- serum lipids.

Risks and side-effects

Prostatic disease

- Androgens stimulate prostatic growth, and testosterone replacement therapy may therefore induce symptoms of bladder outflow obstruction in men with prostatic hypertrophy.
- It is unlikely that testosterone increases the risk of developing prostate cancer but it may promote the growth of an existing cancer.

Polycythaemia

- Testosterone stimulates erythropoiesis. Androgen replacement therapy may increase haemoglobin levels, particularly in older men. It may be necessary to reduce the dose of testosterone in men with clinically significant polycythaemia.

Cardiovascular disease

- Testosterone replacement therapy may cause a fall in both LDL and HDL cholesterol levels, the significance of which remains unclear. The effect of androgen replacement therapy on the risk of developing coronary heart disease is unknown.

Other

- *Acne*
- *Gynaecomastia* is occasionally enhanced by testosterone therapy, particularly in peripubertal boys. This is the result of the conversion of testosterone to oestrogens.
- *Fluid retention* may result in worsening symptoms in those with underlying congestive cardiac failure or hepatic cirrhosis.
- *Obstructive sleep apnoea* may be exacerbated by testosterone therapy.
- *Hepatotoxicity* may be induced by oral androgens, particularly the 17α alkylated testosterones.
- *Mood swings.*

Further reading

Matsumoto AM. Hormonal therapy of male hypogonadism. *Endocrinology and Metabolism Clinics of North America* 1994; 23(4): 857–874.

Tenover JL. Male hormone replacement therapy. *Endocrinology and Metabolism Clinics of North America* 1998; 27(4):969–987.

Table 63.2 Testosterone preparations

Preparation	Dose	Advantage	Problems
Intramuscular testosterone esters	250 mg every 2–3 weeks Monitor pre-dose serum testosterone (should be above the lower limit of normal)	2–3 weekly dosage Effective	I/m injection Wide variations in serum testosterone levels between injections which may be associated with symptoms
Testosterone implants	200–600 mg every 3–6 months Monitor predose serum testosterone	Physiological testosterone levels achieved 3–6 monthly dosing	Minor surgical procedure Risk of infection and pellet extrusion Must remove pellet surgically if complications develop
Transdermal non-scrotal	2.5–7.5 mg daily Monitor testosterone 8 hours after application	Physiological testosterone levels achieved	Skin reactions common
Oral, e.g. testosterone undecanoate and mesterolone (analogue of DHT)	40 mg 3x daily 25 mg 3x daily	Oral preparation	Highly variable efficacy and bioavailability Rarely achieves therapeutic efficacy Multiple daily dosing 17α-alkylated testosterones are not used because of the risk of hepatotoxicity
Transdermal scrotal	4–6 mg daily	Physiological testosterone levels achieved	Supraphysiological levels of DHT may be associated with BPH Unacceptibility of wearing scrotal patch Testosterone levels depend on skin preparation

Chapter 64
Gynaecomastia

Definition

Enlargement of the male breast as a result of hyperplasia of the glandular tissue to a diameter of >2 cm. Common, present in up to 1/3 of men <30 years and in up to 50% of men >45 years.

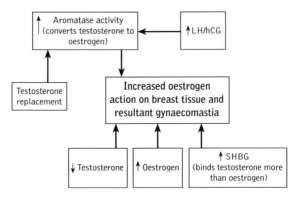

Fig. 64.1 Hormonal influences on gynaecomastia.

Table 64.1 Causes of gynaecomastia

Physiological	Neonatal
	Puberty
	Familial
	Idiopathic
Drugs[a]	Oestrogens, anti-androgens, testosterone
	Spironolactone, ACE inhibitors, calcium antagonists, digoxin
	Alkylating agents
	Alcohol, marijuana, heroin, methadone
	Cimetidine
	Ketoconazole, metronidazole, antituberculous agents
	Tricyclic antidepressants, dopamine antagonists, opiates, benzodiazepines
Hypogonadism	Primary (p. 432)
	Secondary (p. 428)
Tumours	Oestrogen- or androgen-producing testicular or adrenal tumours
	hCG-producing tumours, usually testicular, e.g. germinoma; occasionally ectopic, e.g. lung
	Aromatase-producing testicular tumours
Endocrine	Thyrotoxicosis
	Cushing's syndrome
	Acromegaly
	Androgen insensitivity syndromes
Systemic illness	Liver cirrhosis
	Chronic renal failure
	HIV infection
Other	Chest wall trauma
	Herpes zoster of the chest wall
	Obesity

[a] Possible mechanisms: oestrogen containing, androgen receptor blockers, inhibiting androgen production.

Evaluation

History

- Duration and progression of gynaecomastia.
- Further investigation warranted if:
  - rapidly enlarging gynaecomastia
  - recent onset gynaecomastia in a lean postpubertal man
  - painful gynaecomastia.
- *Exclude underlying tumour*, e.g. testicular cancer.

Symptoms of hypogonadism reduced libido, erectile dysfunction, infertility.

Symptoms of systemic disease e.g. hepatic, renal, and endocrine disease.

Drug history including recreational drugs, e.g. alcohol.

Physical examination

- *Breasts*:
  - Pinch breast tissue between thumb and forefinger – distinguish from fat.
  - Measure glandular tissue diameter. Gynaecomastia if >2 cm.
  - If >5 cm, hard, or irregular, investigate further.
  - Look for galactorrhoea.
- *Testicular palpation:*
  - exclude tumour
  - assess testicular size – ?atrophy.
- *Secondary sex characteristics*
- Look for evidence of *systemic disease* e.g. chronic liver or renal disease, thyrotoxicosis, Cushing's syndrome, chronic cardiac or pulmonary disease

Investigations

Baseline investigations

- serum testosterone
- serum oestradiol
- LH and FSH
- prolactin
- SHBG
- hCG
- liver function tests

Additional investigations

- If testicular tumour is suspected, e.g. raised oestradiol/hCG: testicular ultrasound
- If adrenal tumour is suspected, e.g. markedly raised oestradiol: dehydroepiandrosterone sulfate; abdominal CT or MRI scan.
- If breast malignancy is suspected: mammography; FNAC/tissue biopsy
- If lung cancer is suspected, e.g. raised hCG: chest radiograph

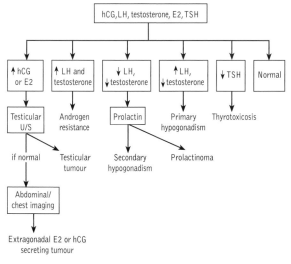

Fig. 64.2 Investigation of gynaecomastia.

Management

- Treat underlying disorder when present. Withdraw offending drugs where possible.
- Reassurance in the majority of idiopathic cases. Often resolves spontaneously.
- Treatment may be required for cosmetic reasons or to alleviate pain.
- Drug treatment rarely effective

Medical
See Table 64.2.

Surgical
Reduction mammoplasty may be required in men with severe and persistent gynaecomastia.

Table 64.2 Medical treatment of gynaecomastia

Drug	Dose (mg/day)	Comments
Tamoxifen	10–30	Antioestrogenic effects. Particularly effective in reducing pain and swelling if used in gynaecomastia of recent onset
Clomiphene	50–100	Antioestrogenic. Reported to be effective in reducing breast size in pubertal gynaecomastia
Testolactone	450	Aromatase inhibitor. Also effective in reducing pubertal gynaecomastia
Danazol	300–600	Non-aromatizable androgen. May also reduce breast size in adults

Chapter 65
Erectile dysfunction

Definition

The consistent inability to acheive or maintain an erect penis sufficient for satisfactory sexual intercourse. Common, present in approximately 10% of males and in >50% of men >70 years.

Physiology of male sexual function

- The erectile response is the result of the coordinated interaction of nerves, smooth muscle of the corpora cavernosa, pelvic muscles and blood vessels.
- It is initiated by psychogenic stimuli from the brain or physical stimulation of the genitalia, which are modulated in the limbic system, transmitted down the spinal cord to the sympathetic and parasympathetic outflows of the penile tissue.
- Penile erectile tissue consists of paired corpora cavernosa on the dorsum of the penis and the corpus spongiosum. These are surrounded by fibrous tissue known as the tunica albuginea.
- In the flaccid state, the corporeal smooth muscle is contracted, minimizing corporeal blood flow and enhancing venous drainage.
- Activation of the erectile pathway results in penile smooth muscle relaxation and cavernosal arterial vasodilatation. As the corporeal sinuses fill with blood, the draining venules are compressed against the tunica albuginea so venous outflow is impaired. This results in penile rigidity and an erection.
- Corporeal vasodilatation is mediated by parasympathetic neuronal activation, which induces nitric oxide release by the cavernosal nerves. This activates guanyl cyclase, thereby increasing cGMP, and causing smooth muscle relaxation.
- Detumescence occurs after the inactivation of cGMP by the enzyme phosphodiesterase, resulting in smooth muscle contraction and vasoconstriction.
- Ejaculation is mediated by the sympathetic nervous system.

Pathophysiology

Erectile dysfunction may thus occur as a result of several mechanisms:

* neurological damage
* arterial insufficiency
* venous incompetence
* androgen deficiency
* penile abnormalities.

Evaluation

History

Sexual history

- Extent of the dysfunction, its duration and progression.
- Presence of nocturnal or morning erections.
- Abrupt onset of erectile dysfunction which is intermittent is often psychogenic in origin.
- Progressive and persistent dysfunction indicates an organic cause.

Symptoms of hypogonadism

- Reduced libido, muscle strength and sense of well-being

Full medical history

- E.g. diabetes mellitus, liver cirrhosis, neurological, cardiovascular or endocrine disease.
- Intermittent claudication suggests a vascular cause.
- A history of genitourinary trauma or surgery is also important.
- Recent change in bladder or bowel function may indicate neurological cause.
- Psychological history.

Drug history

- Onset of impotence in relation to commencing a new medication

Social history

- Stress
- Relationship history
- Recreational drugs including alcohol.

Physical examination

- Evidence of primary or secondary hypogonadism
- Evidence of endocrine disorders
  - hyperprolactinaemia, thyroid dysfunction, hypopituitarism
  - other complications of diabetes mellitus, if present

Table 65.1 Causes of erectile dysfunction

Psychological (20%)	Stress, anxiety
	Psychiatric illness
Drugs (25%)	Alcohol
	Antihypertensives, e.g.diuretics, ß-blockers, methyldopa
	Cimetidine
	Marijuana, heroin, methadone
	Major tranquillizers
	Tricyclic antidepressants, benzodiazepines
	Digoxin
	Glucocorticoids, anabolic steroids
	Oestrogens, antiandrogens
Endocrine (20%)	Hypogonadism (primary or secondary)
	Hyperprolactinaemia
	Diabetes mellitus (30–50% of men with DM >6 years)
	Thyroid dysfunction
Neurological	Spinal cord disorders
	Peripheral and autonomic neuropathies
	Multiple sclerosis
Vascular	Peripheral vascular disease
	Trauma
	Diabetes mellitus
	Venous incompetence
Other	Haemochromatosis
	Debilitating diseases
	Penile abnormalities, e.g. priapism, Peyronie's disease
	Prostatectomy

- Evidence of neurological disease
  - autonomic or peripheral neuropathy
  - spinal cord lesions
- Evidence of systemic disease, e.g.:
  - chronic liver disease
  - chronic cardiac disease
  - peripheral vascular disease
- Genital examination
  - assess testicular size – ?atrophy
  - penile abnormalities, e.g. Peyronie's disease.

Investigation of erectile dysfunction

Baseline investigations

- serum testosterone
- prolactin
- fasting blood glucose
- LH and FSH
- thyroid function tests
- liver function tests
- renal function
- serum lipids
- serum ferritin.

Additional investigations

Rarely required. To assess vascular causes of impotence if corrective surgery is contemplated:

- *Intracavernosal injection* of a vasodilator, e.g. prostaglandin E1 or papaverine. A sustained erection excludes significant vascular insufficiency.
- *Penile doppler ultrasonography* Cavernous arterial flow and venous insufficiency are assessed.

Management

Treat underlying disorder or withdraw offending drugs where possible.

Medical

Androgens

This should be first line therapy in men with hypogonadism (see page 440). Hyperprolactinaemia, when present, should be treated with dopamine agonists and the underlying cause of hypogonadism treated.

Sildenafil (see table 65.2)

Oral phosphodiesterase inhibitor. Acts by enhancing cGMP activity in erectile tissue, thereby amplifying the vasodilatory action of nitric oxide and thus the normal erectile response to sexual stimulation. Only effective following sexual arousal.

* Trials indicate a 70–80% success rate.
* *Dose* 50–100 mg 1 h before sexual activity and no more than once a day. In elderly men and those with renal or hepatic impairment, use 25 mg.

Intracavernous injection

* 70–100% success rate, highest in men with non-vasculogenic impotence.
* Prostaglandin E1 is a potent vasodilator. The dose should be titrated in 1 μg increments until the desired effect is achieved in order to minimize side-effects.
* Papaverine, a phosphodiesterase inhibitor, induces cavernosal vasodilatation and penile rigidity but causes more side-effects.
* *Side-effects*
  – Priapism in 1–5%. Patients must seek urgent medical advice if an erection lasts >4 h.
  – Fibrosis in the injection site in up to 5% of patients. Minimize risk by alternating sides of the penis for injection and injecting a maximum of twice a week.
  – Infection at injection site is rare.
* *Contraindication* Sickle cell disease
* *Injection technique* Avoid the midline so as to avoid urethral and neurovascular damage. Clean the injection site, hold the penis under slight tension and introduce the needle at 90°. Inject after the

Table 65.2 Sildenafil (Viagra), 50 mg

Selective inhibitor of phosphodiesterase type 5	
→ prolonged cyclic GMP activity	
↑ vasodilatory actions of NO on cavernosal smooth muscle	
Contraindications	Recent MI/stroke
	Unstable angina
	Current nitrate use, including isosorbide mononitrate/GTN
	Hypotension (<90/60 mmHg)
	Severe heart failure
	Severe hepatic impairment
	Retinitis pigmentosa
Caution	Hypertension
	Heart disease
	Peyronie's disease
	Sickle cell anaemia
	Leukaemia
	Multiple myeloma
	Bleeding disorders, e.g. active peptic ulcer disease
Ketoconazole HIV protease inhibitors	Indinavir, nelfinavir, saquinavir – start with 25 mg sildenafil (inhibit cytochrome enzyme to give ↑ levels)
Adverse effects	Headaches (16%)
	Facial flushing (19%)
	Dyspepsia (7%)
	Nasal congestion
	Prolonged erection and priapism
	Eye disorders – temporary loss of vision, ↑ ocular pressure, green/blue vision, photosensitivity, blurred vision
	MI
	Ventricular arrhythmia
	Sudden death – mostly in men with pre-existing cardiovascular risk factors

characteristic 'give' of piercing the fibrous capsule. Apply pressure to injection site after removing the needle to prevent bruising.

Vacuum device

• Results are good, with 90% of men achieving a satisfactory erection. The flaccid penis is put into the device and air is withdrawn, creating a vacuum which then allows blood to flow into the penis. A constriction band is then placed on to the base of the penis so that the erection is maintained. This should be removed within 30 min.

• *Side-effects* pain, haematoma.

Penile prosthesis

• Is usually tried in men either reluctant to try other forms of therapy or when other treatments have failed. They may be semi-rigid or inflatable.

• *Complications* infection, mechanical failure.

Psychosexual counselling

• Particularly for men with psychogenic impotence and in men who fail to improve with the above therapies.

Surgical

• Rarely indicated as results are generally disappointing.

• Revascularization techniques may be available in specialist centres.

• Ligation of dorsal veins may restore erectile function temporarily in men with venous insufficiency, although rarely permanently.

Further reading

Cohan P and Korenman SG (2001). Erectile dysfunction. *Journal of Clinical Endocrinology and Metabolism* 86: 2391–2394.

Korenman SG (1998) Sexual function and dysfunction. In Wilson JD, Foster DW, Kronenberg HM, Larson PR (ed.), *William's Textbook of Endocrinology*, 9th edn, pp. 927–938. WB Saunders, Philadelphia.

Sildenafil for erectile dysfunction. *Drugs and Therapeutics Bulletin* 1998; 36(11): 81–83.

Chapter 66
Testicular tumours

Epidemiology

Incidence rising. Currently 6/100 000 men per year.

Risk factors

* cryptorchidism
* gonadal dysgenesis
* infertility/reduced spermatogenesis.

Table 66.1 Classification of testicular tumours

Tumours		Tumour markers
Germ cell tumours (95%)	Seminoma	None
	Non-seminoma	hCG, α-fetoprotein, CEA
	Mixed	
Stromal tumours (2%)	Leydig cell	
	Sertoli cell	
Gonadoblastoma (2%)		
Other (1%)	Lymphoma	
	Carcinoid	

Prognosis

Seminomas

- 95% cure for early disease. 80% cure for stages II/IV.
- Increased incidence of second tumours and leukaemias 20 years after therapy.

Non-seminoma germ cell tumours

- 90% cure in early disease, falling to 60% in metastatic disease.
- Increased incidence of second tumours and leukaemias 20 years after therapy.

Stromal tumours

- Excellent prognosis for benign tumours.
- Malignant tumours are aggressive and are poorly responsive to treatment.

Further reading

Griffin JE, Wilson JD (1998) Disorders of the testes and male reproductive tract. In Wilson JD, Foster DW, Kronenberg HM, Larson PR (ed.), *William's Textbook of Endocrinology*, 9th edn, pp. 819–876. WB Saunders, Philadelphia.

Matsumoto AM (1992) The testis and male sexual function. In Wyngaarden JB, Smith LH, Bennett JC (ed.) *Cecil's Textbook of Medicine*, 19th edn., pp. 1333–1350. WB Saunders, Philadelphia.

Chapter 67
Infertility

Definition

Infertility is defined as failure of pregnancy after 1 year of unprotected regular (2× week) sexual intercourse. It affects 10–15% of all couples.

Causes

- female factors (eg PCOS, tubal damage)   35%
- male factors (idiopathic gonadal failure in 60%)   30%
- combined factors   20%
- unexplained infertility   15%.

Causes of female infertility
- Anovulation
  - PCOS
  - secondary hypogonadism
  - hyperprolactinaemia
  - hypothalamic disease
  - pituitary disease
  - systemic illness
  - drugs, e.g. anabolic steroids
  - POF
- Tubal disorders
  - infective, e.g. chlamydia
  - endometriosis
  - surgery
- Cervical mucus defects
  - Autoimmune
- Uterine abnormalities
  - congenital
  - intrauterine adhesions
  - uterine fibroids.

Causes of male infertility

* Primary gonadal failure
  - genetic Klinefelter's syndrome, Y chromosome deletions, others, e.g. immotile cilia, cystic fibrosis
  - congenital cryptorchidism
  - orchitis
  - torsion or trauma
  - chemotherapy and radiotherapy
  - other toxins, e.g. alcohol, anabolic steroids
  - varicocoele
  - idiopathic
* Secondary gonadal failure
  - Kallman's syndrome (p. 428)
  - IHH
  - structural hypothalamic/pituitary disease
* Genital tract abnormalities
  - obstructive congenital, infective, postsurgical
  - sperm autoimmunity
* Erectile dysfunction
* drugs e.g. spironolactone, corticosteroids, sulfasalazine
* systemic disease e.g. cystic fibrosis, Crohn's disease, and other chronic debilitating diseases.

Evaluation

Sexual history

- *Frequency of intercourse* Infrequent intercourse may reduce sperm quality.
- *Timing of intercourse* Ideal timing is 1–2 days before or after ovulation.
- *Use of lubricants* Should be avoided because of the detrimental effect on semen quality.

Female factors

History

- *Age* Fertility declines rapidly after the age of 36 years.
- *Menstrual history*
  - age at menarche
  - length of menstrual cycle and its predictability (e.g. oligo/amenorrhoea)
  - presence or absence of intermenstrual spotting.
- *Hot flushes* may be indicative of oestrogen deficiency.
- *Spontaneous galactorrhoea* may be caused by hyperprolactinaemia
- *Hypothalamic hypogonadism* suggested by excessive physical exercise (e.g. running >4 miles/day) or weight loss in excess of 10% in 1 year.
- *Drug history*
  - drugs which may cause hyperprolactinaemia (see p. 137), including cocaine and marijuana
  - the use of anabolic steroids may cause secondary hypogonadism
  - cytotoxic chemotherapy or radiotherapy may cause ovarian failure.
- *Medical history* diabetes mellitus, thyroid or pituitary dysfunction, and other systemic illnesses.
- Exclude *tubal disease*
  - recurrent vaginal or urinary tract infections may predispose to pelvic inflammatory disease (PID)
  - dyspareunia and dysmenorrhoea are often present
  - sexually transmitted disease and previous abdominal or gynaecological surgery all predispose to fallopian tube obstruction.

• *Secondary infertility* Details of previous pregnancies including abortions (spontaneous and therapeutic) and ectopic pregnancies should be ascertained.

Physical examination

• *Body mass index* (BMI) The ideal BMI for fertility is 19–24.
• *Secondary sexual characteristics* If absent, look for evidence of Turner's syndrome.
• *Hyperandrogenism* PCOS
• *Galactorrhoea* hyperprolactinaemia
• *External genitalia and pelvic examination.*

Investigations

See Fig. 67.1.

• *Assess ovulatory function*
  – In women with regular menstrual cycles – basal body temperature chart for 2–3 months. A sustained 0.5°C rise in body temperature in the luteal phase (latter half of the menstrual cycle) suggests ovulation. A midluteal (day 21) progesterone (day 1 = first day of menses) should also be measured for confirmation.
  – In women with oligomenorrhoea, check serum FSH, LH, oestradiol, and prolactin.
• *Karyotype* If primary ovarian failure is present (FSH, LH)
• *Serum testosterone, androstenedione and 17α hydroxyprogesterone* if there is clinical evidence of hyperandrogenism.
• *MRI of the pituitary fossa* in hyperprolactinaemia and hypogonadotropic hypogonadism.
• *TSH, free T₄* to exclude thyroid disorders
• *Exclude cervical infection* send vaginal discharge for bacteriology and do chlamydia trachomatis serology
• *Pelvic ultrasound* assess uterine and ovarian anatomy
• *Assess tubal patency*
  – hysterosalpingography (HSG) or laparoscopy (do in the early follicular phase of cycle to avoid doing during pregnancy)
  – should be performed in ovulatory women with a partner who has a normal semen analysis.
• *Further investigations* to be performed if anovulation, male and tubal factors have been excluded as a cause of infertility.
  – *Postcoital test (PCT)* is used to assess cervical mucus receptivity to sperm penetration. Should be performed when mucus is of acceptable quality and quantity (i.e. just before ovulation), and infection and sperm disorders should be excluded prior to

interpretation of results. If PCT is abnormal, then test cervical secretion for antisperm antibodies. Rarely done.

– If there is a past history of recurrent spontaneous abortions, then the presence of *anticardiolipin antibody* should be looked for.

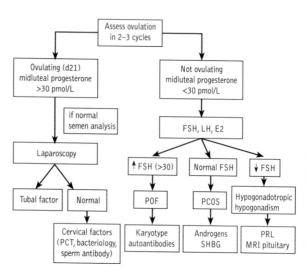

Fig. 67.1 Investigation of female infertility

Male factors

History and physical examination

- *Symptoms of androgen deficiency*
  - reduced libido and potency
  - reduced frequency of shaving
  - may be asymptomatic.
- *Drug history*
  - drug or alcohol abuse and the use of anabolic steroids may all contribute to hypogonadism
  - cytotoxic chemotherapy may cause primary testicular failure.
- *History of infection* e.g. mumps, orchitis, sexually transmitted disease or epididymitis.
- *Bronchiectasis* may be associated with epididymal obstruction (Young's syndrome) or severe aesthenospermia (immotile cilia syndrome).
- *Testicular injury or surgery* may cause disordered spermatogenesis.
- *Secondary sex characteristics* may be absent in congenital hypogonadism.
- *Anosmia* Kallmann's syndrome
- *Eunuchoid habitus* (see p. 435) suggestive of prepubertal hypogonadism.
- *Gynaecomastia* may suggest hypogonadism.
- *Testicular size* (using orchidometer)
  - normal 15–25 ml
  - reduced to <15 ml in hypogonadism
  - in Klinefelter's syndrome, they are often <5 ml.
  - in patients with normal testicular size, suspect genital tract obstruction, e.g. congenital absence of vas deferens.
- Examine rest of *external genitalia* look for penile/urethral abnormalities and epididymal thickening.

Investigations

Semen analysis

Essential in the diagnostic work up of any infertile couple.

- If *normal* (see table 67.1) then a male cause is excluded and the test does not have to be repeated.
- If *abnormal*, then repeat semen analysis 6–12 weeks later.
- Semen collection should be performed after 3 days of sexual abstinence. See Table 67.1 for interpretation of results.
- If *azoospermia* is present, then obstruction is ruled out by normal FSH and testosterone concentrations.
- *Asthenospermia*, or immotile sperm, is usually due to immunological infertility or infection, e.g. of the prostate (high semen viscosity and pH, and leukocytospermia)

FSH, LH, and testosterone levels

- FSH may be elevated in the presence of normal LH and testosterone levels and oligospermia. This may be seen in men who are normally virilized but infertile as a result of disordered spermatogenesis.
- Low FSH, LH and testosterone concentrations suggest secondary hypogonadism. An MRI of the pituitary gland and hypothalamus is necessary to exclude organic disease.

Further investigations

- *Urinary bacteriology* should be performed in men with leukocytospermia.
- *Sperm antibodies* in blood and semen should also be measured in most infertile men.
- *Scrotal ultrasound* may help in the diagnosis of chronic epididymitis. Men being investigated for infertility are at increased risk of testicular tumours.
- *Karyotyping* may be helpful in men with primary testicular failure. Klinefelter's syndrome (47,XXY) is a common cause of infertility, and deletions on the long arm of the Y chromosome have been found in a significant proportion of azoospermic males.
- *Testicular biopsy* is rarely diagnostic, but may be used to retrieve sperm for assisted reproduction techniques in men with obstructive azoospermia.
- *Sperm function tests* are rarely required, but may be used to predict ability of sperm to fertilize human oocytes.

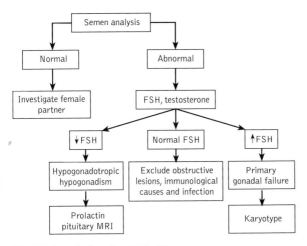

Fig. 67.2 Investigation of male infertility.

Table 67.1 WHO criteria for normal semen analysis

Test	Normal values	Nomenclature for abnormal values
Volume	2–6 ml	Aspermia (no ejaculate)
pH	7.2–8	
Sperm concentration	>20 × 10⁶/ml	Oligozoospermia
Total sperm count	>40 × 10⁶/ejaculate	Azoospermia (no sperm in ejaculate)
Motility	>50%	Asthenospermia
Morphology	>30% normal forms	Teratospermia
Live sperm	>70%	Necrospermia
Leukocytes	<1 × 10⁶/ml	Leukocytospermia
Immunobead test (for sperm antibodies)	<20% spermatozoa with adherent particles	

(from Guzick *et al. NEJM*, 2001, 345: 1388–93.)

Management

Female partner

Anovulation

- *Normogonadotrophic*
  - usually PCOS: weight reduction if obese
  - ovulation induction (see p. 479).
- *Hypergonadotrophic*
  - *POF* ovum donation followed by IVF is only option.
  - spontaneous transient remission possible in early POF
  - if still cycling and FSH 15–25IU/L, ovarian hyperstimulation and IVF may be attempted, but poor results.
- *Hypogonadotrophic*
  - if hyperprolactinaemic then dopamine agonists are usually effective
  - lifestyle changes if underweight/excessive exercise
  - otherwise, ovulation induction (see p. 479).

Tubal infertility

- Surgical tubal reconstruction may be attempted.
- 50–60% 2 year cumulative pregnancy rate in patients with mild disease, but only 10% in more severe disease and high risk of ectopic pregnancy, so IVF better in most cases.
- Cumulative pregnancy rate at least 50% following IVF (20–25% per cycle) unless hydrosalpinx is present, in which case the pregnancy rate is halved.

Endometriosis

- *Minimal/mild*
  - GnRH agonists, danazol, and progestagens are ineffective
  - laparoscopic destruction of superficial disease improves pregnancy chances slightly.
  - assisted reproductive techniques (ART) (p. 475) give pregnancy rate of 25–35% per cycle.
- *Severe* (tubal obstruction ovarian involvement) Surgery. However, ART often necessary.

Table 67.2 Assisted reproduction techniques (ART)

Technique	Indications	Pregnancy rates	Notes
Intrauterine insemination (IUI)	Unexplained infertility Mild oligozoospermia ($>2 \times 10^6$ motile sperm) Immunological factors	50% after 3 cycles	hMG and hCG are used to induce superovulation. Prepared spermatozoa are then injected into the uterine cavity through a catheter 12 h after ovulation Ineffective if severe male factor, endometriosis, or tubal damage
In vitro fertilization (IVF)	Most forms of infertility unless severe male factor	25% pregnancy rate per cycle 80–90% delivery rate after 6 cycles in women under the age of 35 years Success rates markedly reduced >40 years of age	After superovulation, ovarian follicles are aspirated under ultrasonic guidance and are fertilized with prepared sperm in vitro. The embryos are then transferred back into the uterine cavity, usually 48 h after aspiration May adopt a similar technique in women with premature ovarian failure, using donated ova which are then fertilized in vitro with partner's sperm. Hormonal support will be required following embryo transfer. Cumulative pregnancy rate of 50–60%

Table 67.2 *contid.*

Technique	Indications	Pregnancy rates	Notes
Gamete intrafallopian transfer (GIFT)	Most forms of infertility unless severe male factor Do not use in women with tubal disease	Similar to IVF	Similar to IVF except that retrieved follicles and sperm are injected laparoscopically into a fallopian tube to fertilize naturally
Intracytoplasmic sperm injection (ICSI)	Male infertility	20% per cycle if female partner <40 years of age	Spermatozoa injected directly into oocytes retrieved following superovulation. Embryos are then implanted into the uterus. Spermatozoa may be concentrated from an ejaculate or be aspirated from the epididymis or testis in men with obstructive azoospermia Small risk of sex chromosome abnormalities in males (1%) conceived following ICSI

Vaginal/cervical factors

* *Infection* Each episode of acute PID causes infertility in 10–15% of cases. Chlamydia trachomatis is responsible for half the cases of PID in the developed countries. Treat both partners with antibiotics.
* *Immunological* Intruterine insemination (IUI) ± superovulation. If this fails, then ART.

Male partner

Hypogonadotrophic hypogonadism

* Gonadotrophins: hCG 1000–2000 IU i/m 2–3x week. Most also require FSH/hMG 75–150 IU i/m 3x week. Main side-effect: gynaecomastia.

or

* Pulsatile GnRH using a subcutaneous infusion pump (see p. 481). Dose varies from 25–600 ng/kg every 90–120 min. Titrate to normalize LH, FSH, and testosterone. Will not work in pituitary disease.
* Once testes are >8 ml, semen analysis every 6 months. Takes at least 2 years to maximize spermatogenesis. 30% of couples will achieve pregnancy.

Obstructive azoospermia

Microsurgery possible, but better results with ICSI.

Varicocoele

Controversial association with male subfertility. Treat in adolescents if affected testis reduced by 3 ml compared with other testes, and in young infertile couples (<30 years) of <3 years infertility if subnormal semen analysis.

Unexplained infertility

Definition

Infertility despite normal sexual intercourse occurring at least twice weekly, normal semen analysis, documentation of ovulation in several cycles, and normal laparoscopy.

Management

30% will become pregnant within 3 years of expectant management. If not pregnant by then, chances that spontaneous pregnancy will occur are greatly reduced and ART should be considered. In women >30 years of age then expectant management is not an option and superovulation + IUI or IVF should be considered.

Results

- IUI can acheive a pregnancy rate of 15% per cycle and cumulative delivery rate after several cycles = 50%.

- IVF offers a pregnancy rate of 25% per cycle and a cumulative delivery rate approaching 80%. Significant risk of multiple pregnancy with any form of ART.

Ovulation induction

Indications

* Anovulation due to:
  – polycystic ovary syndrome
  – hypopituitarism
  – hypogonadotrophic hypogonadism
* Controlled ovarian hyperstimulation for ART.

Pretreatment assessment

* Exclude thyroid dysfunction and hyperprolactinaemia.
* Check rubella serology.
* Confirm normal semen analysis.
* Confirm tubal patency (laparoscopy) prior to gonadotrophin use and/or after failed clomiphene use.
* Optimize lifestyle: maintain satisfactory BMI, exercise in moderation, reduce alcohol intake and stop smoking.
* Baseline pelvic ultrasound is essential to exclude ovarian masses and uterine abnormalities prior to treatment.

Clomiphene citrate

* *Mode of action*
  – binds to oestrogen receptors in hypothalamus, blocking normal –ve feedback thereby increasing pulse frequency of GnRH. This stimulates FSH and LH release
  – antioestrogen effect on endometrium, cervix, and vagina.
* *Indications* eugonadotropic anovulation, e.g. PCOS. Requires normal hypothalamo–pituitary–ovarian axis to work therefore ineffective in hypogonadotrophic hypogonadism.
* *Contraindications* hepatic dysfunction
* *Administration*   Start on days 2–5 of menstrual cycle (may have to induce bleed by giving a progestagen for 10 days) and take for a total of 5 days.
* *Dose*
  – start on 25–50 mg/day and increase by 50 mg every month until midluteal progesterone is >30 nmol/L
  – spontaneous ovulation should occur 5–10 days after last day of medication

- remain on optimum dose for 3–6 months
- most require 50–100 mg/day
- Some centres advocate regular vaginal ultrasound to monitor follicle growth.

- *Efficacy*
  - 80–90% ovulate, with conception rates of 50–60% in first 6 ovulatory cycles. May enhance chances of ovulation in non-responders by the administration of 10 000 IU of hCG midcycle (use ultrasound guidance; administer hCG when leading follicle is at least 20 mm).
  - In hyperandrogenic women, particularly adult onset CAH, addition of dexamethasone 0.5 mg at night may improve success rates.

- *Side-effects*
  - hot flushes in 10%, mood swings, depression and headaches in 1%, pelvic pain in 5%, nausea in 2%, breast tenderness in 5%, hair loss in 0.3%, visual disturbances in 1.5%
  - mild OHSS in 5%
  - multiple pregnancies in 10%.

- *Risk of ovarian cancer* Unknown. Infertility is associated with an increased risk of ovarian cancer. Additionally, one study suggests a twofold increased risk of low grade ovarian cancer following long-term clomiphene use. Further studies necessary but currently recommended maximum treatment duration is 6 months.

Gonadotrophins

- *Indications*
  - hypogonadotrophic hypogonadism
  - women with PCOS who are clomiphene resistant.
  - in combination with IUI in unexplained infertility
  - for superovulation as part of ART.

- *Dose and administration* Several regimes available, all require close monitoring with twice weekly oestradiol (E2) measurements and vaginal ultrasounds. One suggested regime (low dose step-up approach):
  - Start at 50–75IU/day hMG (or FSH) on day 2–4 of the menstrual cycle. On day 7 of treatment measure serum E2 and perform a vaginal ultrasound. If E2 <200 pmol/L and there has been no change in follicle development then increase hMG (or FSH) to 75–112 IU/day.
  - If >3 mature follicles (>14 mm) develop or E2 >3000 pmol/L then abandon cycle and restart on half-dose hMG/FSH because of risk of OHSS.

- Otherwise, give hCG at a dose of 5000 IU to trigger ovulation when follicle >18 mm diameter. May increase to 10 000 IU in subsequent cycle if ovulation doesn't occur.
- May use gonadotrophins for a total of 6 cycles. If unsuccessful then consider ART.

- *Efficacy* 80–85% pregnancy rate after 6 cycles.

- *Side-effects*
  - multiple pregnancy (20%)
  - OHSS.

- *Ovarian hyperstimulation syndrome* (OHSS)

- A syndrome of ovarian enlargement and increased vascular permeability with accumulation of fluid in the peritoneal, pleural and pericardial cavities. Occurs during the luteal phase of the cycle, i.e. after hCG stimulation and is more severe if pregnancy occurs due to endogenous hCG production.

- Mild OHSS occurs in up to 25% of stimulated cycles and results in abdominal bloating and nausea. It resolves with bed rest and fluid replacement. Severe OHSS, associated with hypotension, markedly enlarged ovaries, ascites, and pleural and pericardial effusions, occurs in <0.1%. Women need to be hospitalized and resuscitated as there is an increased mortality from disseminated intravascular coagulation and pulmonary emboli.

- OHSS is best prevented by witholding hCG during at-risk cycles.

GnRH treatment

- *Indications* Hypothalamic hypogonadism with normal pituitary function.

- *Dose and administration* Pulsatile GnRH using an infusion pump which is worn continuously. This delivers a dose of GnRH every 90–120 min. The dose may be administered either intravenously (5 μg/90 min) or subcutaneously (20 μg/90 min).

- *Monitoring*
  - monitor E2 levels because risk of hypo-oestrogenaemia if GnRH is given too frequently.
  - no risk of OHSS or multiple pregnancies so ultrasonic monitoring is unnecessary.

- *Side-effects* allergic reaction

- *Efficacy* cumulative pregnancy rate of 80–90%.

Further reading

Forti G, Krausz C. Evaluation and treatment of the infertile couple. *Journal of Clinical Endocrinology and Metabolism* 1998; 83(12): 4177–4188.

Hargreave T, Ghosh C. Male fertility disorders. *Endocrinology and Metabolism Clinics of North America* 1998; 27(4): 765–782.

Hull MGR, Cahill DJ. Female infertility. *Endocrinology and Metabolism Clinics of North America* 1998; 27(4): 851–876.

Chapter 68
Disorders of sexual differentiation

Clinical presentation

• *Infancy* ambiguous genitalia (evaluation is discussed p. 650)
• *Puberty*
  – failure to progress through puberty (male or female phenotype)
  – primary amenorrhoea in a female phenotype
  – virilization of a female phenotype
• *Adulthood*
  – hypogonadism
  – infertility

Evaluation

• *Karyotype* 46,XX vs 46,XY male or female
• Imaging
  – look for presence of testes or ovaries and uterus
  – most easily performed using pelvic ultrasound but MRI may be more sensitive in identifying internal genitalia.

Hormonal evaluation

• LH/FSH
• Testosterone, androstenedione, SHBG
• 17-hydroxyprogesterone ± ACTH stimulation (p. 367)
• hCG stimulation test (p. 437) – to assess the presence of functioning testicular material. Measure testosterone, androstenedione, DHT and SHBG post-stimulation
• Others depending on clinical suspicion, e.g. 5α-reductase deficiency – check DHT levels before and after hCG stimulation.

Causes (see also p. 650)

46,XY – undervirilized male

* Gonadal differentiation abnormalities, e.g. gonadal dysgenesis
  – cause unknown in the majority
  – may result from 45,X/46,XY mosaicism or SRY gene mutation.
* Leydig cell abnormalities
  – autosomal recessive
  – due to inactivating LH receptor gene mutation
* CAH, e.g.
  – 3β-HSD, 17α-hydroxylase/17,20-desmolase or 17β-HSD deficiencies
  – congenital lipoid adrenal hyperplasia (due to StAR gene mutation).
* Androgen receptor defects
  – androgen insensitivity syndrome
* 5α-reductase deficiency
  – mutation of 5α-reductase type 2 gene
  – autosomal recessive inheritance
  – results in high testosterone but low DHT concentrations
* Persistent mullerian duct syndrome
  – mullerian inhibitory substance (MIS) or MIS receptor gene mutation
* True hermaphrodite

46,XX – virilized female

* Excess foetal androgens – CAH
  – 21-OH deficiency (commonest cause)
  – 11β-OH deficiency.
* Excess maternal androgens
  – drugs
  – virilizing tumours
* Placental aromatase deficiency

46,XX males

  – due to a Y to X translocation so that the SRY gene is present
  – phenotype similar to Klinefelter's syndrome
* True hermaphrodite

Androgen insensitivity syndrome

Pathogenesis

+ Results from a defect in androgen receptor number or function. This may be complete or partial. The androgen receptor is on chromosome Xq. Several mutations may occur, inherited in an X-linked recessive fashion. Poor correlation between genotype and phenotype.
+ Rare – 1 : 20 000–1 : 64 000 males.

Clinical features

+ *Complete androgen insensitivity (testicular feminization)* results in normal female external genitalia. No male external sex organs present, but remnants of mullerian structures are occasionally present. Testes abdominal or in the inguinal canal. Vagina often shorter than normal.
+ Often present during puberty with primary amenorrhoea. Height above female average, breast development normal. Little or no pubic and axillary hair. Gender identity is female.
+ *Partial androgen insensitivity* has a wide phenotypic spectrum, ranging from ambiguous genitalia to a normal male phenotype presenting with infertility.
+ 9% risk of seminoma.

Hormonal evaluation

+ Testosterone and androstenedione levels are often above normal. hCG stimulation results in a further rise in testosterone, with little increase in SHBG.
+ Oestradiol levels are higher than in normal males, but lower than the female average. Oestrogen is produced from the aromatization of testosterone.
+ LH levels are usually markedly elevated, but FSH is normal.
+ Genetic testing is possible in some centres.

Management

+ Orchidectomy in adolescence after attaining puberty
+ Oestrogen replacement therapy to induce puberty and continue thereafter

True hermaphroditism

Pathogenesis

- Unknown. May be familial.
- Affected individuals have both ovarian and testicular tissue, either in the same gonad (ovotestis), or an ovary on one side and a testis on the other. A uterus and a fallopian tube are usually present, the latter on the side of the ovary or ovotestis. Wolffian structures may be present in a third of individuals on the side of the testis. The testicular tissue is usually dysgenetic although the ovarian tissue may be normal.

Clinical features

- Most individuals have ambiguous genitalia and are raised as males, but just under 10% have normal female external genitalia.
- At puberty, 50% of individuals menstruate, which may present as cyclic haematuria in males and most develop breasts.
- Feminization and virilization vary widely. Most are infertile, but fertility has been reported.
- 2% risk of gonadal malignancy, higher in 46,XY individuals.

Hormonal evaluation

- 46,XX in 70%, 46,XX/46,XY in 20% and 46,XY in 10%.
- Hypergonadotropic hypogonadism is usual.
- Diagnosis can only be made on gonadal biopsy.

General principles of management

Assignment of gender and reconstructive surgery

Female pseudohermaphroditism

- As these girls are potentially fertile, they should be brought up as female.
- Clitoromegaly is usually corrected in infancy by clitoroplasty. Vaginoplasty is usually deferred until late adolescence. Results of feminizing genitoplasty with regard to sexual activity are promising, albeit variable.

Male pseudohermaphroditism

- The decision regarding gender reassignment is more complex and depends on the degree of sexual ambiguity in addition to the cause of the disorder and the potential for normal sexual function and fertility.
- Individuals with complete androgen insensitivity are assigned a female sex as they are resistant to testosterone therapy, develop female sexual characteristics, and have a female gender identity. They may require vaginaplasty in adolescence.
- Individuals with 5α-reductase deficiency should be raised as males where possible because of subsequent virilization and attainment of male gender identity at puberty.
- Sex assignment of other forms of male pseudohermaphroditism depends on phallic size. If the stretched penile length is >2.5 cm then it is likely that reconstructive surgery will be successful and therefore a male sex may be assigned. A trial of 3 months of testosterone may be used to enhance phallic growth prior to surgery (25–50 mg depot testosterone/month).
- Penile reconstruction and orchidopexy is best performed at about 1 year of age. However, multiple surgery is often required. Testicular prostheses inserted in adolescence may be required if orchidopexy is not possible. Results for sexual function are encouraging, with centres reporting an average of 70% success.

Gonadectomy

- Increased risk of gonadoblastoma in most individuals with abdominal testes. Risk is highest in those with dysgenetic gonads and

Y chromosome material. Bilateral gonadectomy should therefore be performed.

- Optimal timing of the gonadectomy is unknown. In androgen insensitivity, the risk of gonadoblastoma appears to rise only after the age of 20 years so orchidectomy is recommended in adolescence after attaining puberty. In most other disorders, gonadectomy prior to puberty is recommended.

- Early bilateral orchidectomy should also be performed in 46,XY subjects with 5α-reductase deficiency or 17ß HSD deficiency who are being raised as females to prevent virilization at puberty.

Hormone replacement therapy

- Patients with disorders of adrenal biosynthesis, e.g. CAH, require lifelong glucocorticoid and usually mineralocorticoid replacement therapy.

- Most male pseudohermaphrodites and hermaphrodites being raised as male require long-term testosterone replacement therapy.

- Individuals with 5α-reductase deficiency usually receive supra-physiological doses of testosterone in order to achieve satisfactory DHT levels.

- Subjects with androgen insensitivity and male pseudohermaphrodites being raised as female should receive oestrogen replacement therapy to induce puberty and this should be continued thereafter.

Psychological support

- Disorders relating to sexual identity and function often require experienced counselling.

- Patient support groups are often helpful.

Further reading

Simpson JL. Disorders of sexual differentiation. *Current Opinion in Endocrinology and Diabetes* 1996;3: 452–462.

Vogiatzi MG, New MI. Differential diagnosis and therapeutic options for ambiguous genitalia. *Current Opinion in Endocrinology and Diabetes* 1998;5: 3–10.

Warne GL, Zajac JD. Disorders of sexual differentiation. *Endocrinology and Metabolism Clinics of North America* 1998;27(4): 945–967.

Chapter 69
Transsexualism

Definition

A condition in which an anatomically and genetically normal person feels that he or she is a member of the opposite sex. There is an irreversible discomfort with the anatomical gender, which may be severe, often developing in childhood.

Epidemiology

- More common in males.
- Estimated incidence of 1 : 12 000 men and 1 : 30 000 women.

Management

Principles

* Multidisciplinary approach between psychiatrists, endocrinologists and surgeons.
* Endocrine disorders should be excluded prior to entry into the gender reassignment programme – i.e. ensure normal internal and external genitalia, karyotype, gonadotrophins, and testosterone/oestradiol.
* Psychological assessment is essential before definitive therapy. This should take place over at least 2 years to ensure a permanent diagnosis.
* Following this period, the subject is encouraged to cross-gender dress under the supervision of a psychiatrist. This should continue for at least 1 year before hormonal manipulation.
* Psychological follow-up should continue throughout the programme, including after surgery.

Hormonal manipulation

Male to female transsexuals

* Suppress male secondary sex characteristics: cyproterone acetate (CPA) (100 mg/day)
* Induce female secondary sex characteristics: EE2 (100 μg/day)
* *Aims:*
  – breast development – maximum after 1–2 years of treatment
  – development of female fat distribution
  – decreased body hair and smoother skin
  – decreased muscle bulk and strength
  – reduction in testicular size
  – ?effect on behaviour.
* Gradually reduce dose of CPA as testosterone levels fall. May stop CPA following gender reassignment surgery.
* The dose of EE2 may be reduced when there is little further progression in female secondary sex characteristics, usually after 1 year of treatment.
* May then substitute EE2 for conjugated oestrogens or oestradiol valerate, both of which are associated with a lower complication rate.

Gender reassignment surgery

* Performed at least 6–9 months after starting sex hormone therapy
* Usually performed in several stages.

Male to female transsexuals

* bilateral orchidectomy and resection of the penis
* construction of a vagina and labia minora
* clitoroplasty
* breast augmentation.

Female to male transsexuals

* bilateral mastectomy
* hysterectomy and salpingo-oophorectomy
* phalloplasty and testicular prostheses.

Table 69.1 Maintenance doses of oestrogens used in male to female transsexuals

Oestrogen	Daily dose
Ethinyl oestradiol	30–50 μg
Oestradiol valerate (oral)	2–4 mg
Oestradiol valerate (transdermal)	50–100 μg
Conjugated oestrogen	1.25 mg

- Adjust oestrogen dose depending on plasma LH and oestradiol levels (see table 69.1).
- *Side-effects* (particularly while on high dose EE2+CPA therapy):
  - hyperprolactinaemia (EE2 stimulates prolactin synthesis and secretion in addition to inducing proliferation of pituitary lactotrophs)
  - thromboembolism, both arterial and venous
  - abnormal liver enzymes
  - depression
  - ? increased risk of breast cancer.

Female to male transsexuals

- Induce male secondary sex characteristics and suppress female secondary sex characteristics: parenteral testosterone (e.g. Sustanon 250 mg) every 2 weeks.
- *Aims:*
  - cessation of menstrual bleeding
  - atrophy of uterus and breasts
  - increase muscle bulk and strength
  - deepenening of voice
  - hirsutism
  - male body fat distribution
  - increase in libido.
- Once sexual characteristics are stable (after approximately 1 year of treatment), reduce testosterone injection frequency according to serum testosterone levels.
- *Side-effects:*
  - acne
  - weight gain
  - abnormal liver function
  - adverse lipid profile.

Monitoring of therapy

- Every 3 months for first year then every 6 months
- Hormonal therapy is lifelong and so patients should be followed up indefinitely:
  - physical examination
  - liver function tests
  - serum lipids
  - hormonal status (LH, FSH, prolactin, oestradiol, testosterone).

Prognosis

- No increased mortality.
- Increased morbidity in male to female transsexuals from thromboembolism.
- No increased morbidity in female to male transsexuals.
- Hyperprolactinaemia and elevation in liver enzymes are self-limiting in the majority of cases.
- The risk of osteoporosis is not increased in transsexuals.
- There may be a slightly increased risk of breast cancer in male to female transsexuals.
- Results from reconstructive surgery, particularly in female to male transsexuals, remain suboptimal.

Further reading

Schlatterer K, von Werder K, Stalla GK. Multistep treatment concept of transsexual patients. *Experimental and Clinical Endocrinology and Diabetes* 1996; 104: 413–419.

Index